THE
Busy Girl's
HOT
Body Plan

Anthony Punshon

Before we get into the good stuff, let's cover the boring legal stuff! That'll be fun right? (Sorry, it does have to be done!)

DISCLAIMER

The information presented herein is in no way intended as medical advice or to serve as a substitute for medical counselling. Rather, as with all exercise and nutrition programmes, The Busy Girl's Hot Body Plan is intended only to supplement, not replace, medical care or advice as part of a healthful lifestyle. As such, the information should be used in conjunction with the guidance and care of your physician. You must consult your physician before beginning this programme as you would with any exercise and nutrition programme. If you choose not to obtain the consent of your physician and/or work with your physician throughout the duration of your time using The Busy Girl's Hot Body Plan, you are agreeing to accept full responsibility for your actions. By utilising the exercise and nutritional strategies contained herein, you recognise that despite all precautions on the part of Anthony Punshon and PW Physique and Fitness, there are risks of injury or illness which can occur because of your use of the aforementioned information and you expressly assume such risks and waive, relinquish and release any claim which you may have against Anthony Punshon and PW Physique and Fitness, or its affiliates as a result of any future physical injury or illness incurred in connection with, or as a result of, the use or misuse of the exercise and nutritional strategies contained in, associated with, or performed in conjunction with The Busy Girl's Hot Body Plan.

First Edition: December 2017

Published in Great Britain in 2017 by
PW Physique and Fitness
Horton Buildings
Goring Street
Goring-by-sea
West Sussex
BN12 5AD

Photographs by IC Photographics, and Cherry Red Photography

Copyright © Anthony Punshon and PW Physique and Fitness 2017

ISBN: 978-1981311989

Acknowledgements

I always said I wouldn't write another book. As it turns out, I was just waiting for the right book to come out. And this book was only possible because it was a real team effort. So let's start from the front!

The amazing cover photo was shot here in Worthing, and is of **Amelia Carr**. Amelia is the ultimate 'busy girl', owning the hugely successful *Regnante School of Performing Arts (RSOPA)*, so is always on the go and always putting others first because she's not just an incredible woman, but also a beautiful soul.

Her hair was styled by **Josh Treanor** from premier salon Infusion Hair Design, and her make-up was by one of my best friends, **Sonia Martin**, who is the owner of *La Belle Beauty Salon and Training Academy* and serial entrepreneur.

The photo was taken by my other bestie, and ace photographer **Laura Brennan**, owner of *Cherry Red Photography*.

The beautiful faces and hot bodies demonstrating the exercises for you belong to friends and clients **Stacey Church, Laura Thom, Pippa Hickey, Serena Stone**, and **Megan Franklin**, most of whom were captured beautifully by photographer **Sophie Bowden-Caldwell** from *IC Photographics*.

The meals section was made all the more tasty thanks to **Natalie Noble, Glynis Stringer, Nicola Hinton**, and **Pippa Sayer**. All amazing clients walking the walk.

Sara Guiel, co-owner of multi-national networking business *The Mumpreneurs Networking Club* took time out of her insanely busy life to write the foreword, and **Kelie Hoadley, Nicole Parker, Melody Clarke, Gail Waller**, and **Val Gayes** not only changed their lives with the principles in this book, but took he time to share their inspirational stories. **Sophie Bowden-Caldwell** is also responsible for **Kelie, Melody, Gail**, and **Val's** beautiful after photos.

And we're still going...

Gail Waller (overdelivering as always!), **Nicola House**, and **Sue Fenwick** dived in to proof-read big chunks of this on short notice for me before I went into the recording studio to get the first half of the audio-book recorded.

And lastly my incredible, and incredibly understanding fiancée **Nicola Lloyd** who has done everything from proof-read, format, add her favourite meals, and generally made her eyes bleed staring at her laptop screen to make this book possible.

Contents

Part Four: Crank it Up

Part Five: Keep it Up

Foreword

Since time began women have gone about their lives, working, raising children, maintaining households and more often than not wishing they could carve out the time it takes to get that body. You know the one, THAT one. The one that doesn't take up homework supervising time, Grandma's hospital visiting time, or that really important, funding meeting time.

We know it takes planning and action - we're not daft, we know if you put nothing in you get nothing out. We know just wishing we had that body isn't going to cut it, in every other area of our lives we plan and action.

We convene the board and plan corporate expansion, we go to parents' evenings and decide to get a more effective homework plan together, so fast growing teenagers can nail those dreaded exams, we launder our work uniform on a Friday ready for a Monday. We know that actioning a plan is the way forward. So why is our body plan missing from this mix? Why is it not a habitual part of our ever-present juggling?

We know that everyone has 24 hours a day- EVERYONE. You and me, and swimsuit models - 24 hours! We could ditch EastEnders on catch up, we could get up 20 minutes earlier (I know, that doesn't thrill me either- especially in the winter months!) but where would we start? Can we do it? How do we sustain it? If we're going to do that it's got to be absolutely worth it. We're experts at refereeing sibling squabbles, chauffeuring teens or getting to work on time and making a difference in our world of work, volunteering or on the domestic front line. But we're not experts at everything, and sometimes we just need to fess up, and look to an expert!

It's not easy to ask for help when we're so self-reliant in every other area of our lives, making it up and muddling through and mostly hitting and not missing. This is especially true when it feels self-indulgent, we know it's about looking after ourselves, not luxurious fun, but we still feel guilty that it's not work or family. And that's why we need an expert, especially one that can teach us how to take the steps necessary to get that body without putting the brakes on family movie night, or taking the extra shifts to pay for Christmas. I run a national organisation, I have three children and I only have 24 hours a day and no real expertise in nutrition and exercise, certainly none that I haven't learned from Anthony. I managed to somehow fit his advice and instruction in to my schedule - it wasn't easy and sometimes it was more than just a bit tricky, and I tripped up, spent that extra 20 minutes in bed but the grounding this expert gives you means that time and again you can return to it his expertise to reform those habits so that body you wish for, can be a consistent reality.

And now Anthony has written it down for you, for us! An easy guide, he's told us what it takes, where to start, what to do and made the workout time short and powerful. He's done it, tested it, refined it and written the plan so in this one area of your life, this important one, the one where you just don't know where to start but want oh so much to get going if someone would just tell you how - you can! We can read instructions, we're happy to take advice and we'll implement it to get results, after all, we're not daft - we were just waiting for this plan!

Sara Guiel
Director, Mumpreneurs Networking Club

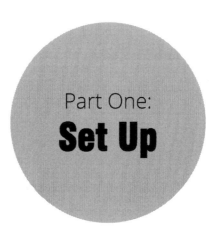

Part One:
Set Up

Chapter 1

Three Truths
That Will Set You
Free

"You can't get rid of it with exercise alone. You can do the most vigorous exercise and only burn up 300 calories in an hour. If you've got fat on your body, the exercise firms and tones the muscles. But when you use that tape measure, what makes it bigger? It's the fat!"

– Jack LaLanne

It's dark. You wake to hear this obnoxious sound cutting through the darkness. You reach out one arm and feel around for your phone so you can shut your alarm off before the noise pushes your brain out of your nostrils.

Before you open your eyes, you quickly have a conversation in your head. *"I don't have to get up now. It was a late night. I can work out after work instead. Or maybe in my lunch hour. If I hit snooze, I could have 8 more minutes sleep. 8 more minutes. Mmmmmm..."*

You snap yourself out of it.

"NO! I'm getting up NOW. Come on. Just put one foot on the floor. Open your eyes. Not too fast... OK, we've got this."

You manage to get yourself to your feet and shuffle out to the kitchen. You've got over the hard bit now. You've dragged yourself out of bed. As long as you can make it to the kettle, you can drag yourself to a workout.

Mission accomplished.

The next morning, it's dark. You wake to hear this obnoxious sound cutting through the darkness. You reach out one arm and feel around for your phone so you can shut your alarm off before the noise pushes your brain out of your nostrils.

The ritual starts again.

You do it though, because if you do, you know you'll get tight abs, hotter curves, and an all-round sexier, healthier you.

So every morning, you fight your alarm, have that conversation in your head, and drag yourself out to the gym or for that run.

Two months later you step out of the shower. You have a little shiver as you step from the steaming hot water into the cold air of your bathroom, then have a little chuckle to yourself for shivering. Still wet you check the mirror. *"Where are my abs, dammit? I must have run a million miles by now, why aren't I cracking walnuts with my butt cheeks?"*

When we make that decision to change and we finally muster up the courage and discipline it takes to drag ourselves to work out on a regular basis, there are common things we overlook, or even sweep under the carpet. Then we run ourselves into the ground for months without seeing significant results, like we're trapped on a hamster wheel. Working hard, but ultimately getting nowhere.

And it's because we don't apply these three rules:

Lean Living Rule #1: You Can't Outrun Your Mouth

When we start a new programme, this is the single biggest thing that we ignore — or bury our heads in the sand hoping it won't apply! And it's not that we don't know that we need to eat better, but it's almost like we take the approach of 'if it's better than how we eat now, it'll be *good enough*'. After all, we can just burn the rest off with exercise, right?

In reality though, eating a bit more fruit and saying "No" to the odd dessert every now and again won't get the job done. Exercise just isn't that effective!

Here's some quick maths:

30 minutes of cardio will burn around 200 calories, give or take. That's roughly the same amount of calories as is in a fancy latte, and I bet getting one of those down would be a lot easier (and quicker)!

But there's something else to consider too. Studies have shown that you won't even touch your fat stores until you've been going for an hour and a half straight! So, to so much as dent your fat stores through exercise, you'd need to do *more* than 90 minutes at a time.

Alrighty then.

If you're serious about getting in shape, you need to get your eating plan in order, plain and simple. Don't rely on exercise to do the job for you. If you put the wrong fuel in your car, it'll go nowhere. Believe me, I've done this! And the same applies to you.

Once you understand and accept this, not only will the fat start dropping off, but because you've removed the thing that was layering the fat on, the bad eating, you'll never see that fat again! And don't worry, in part two I'm going to show you how to make eating for that lean, sexy body easier than falling off a treadmill.

Lean Living Rule #2: Working Out *More* Won't Improve Your Results

If something's good, then more of it must be better, right?

Not so much! In fact, working out too much is not only responsible for stopping eager new exercisers faster than the Diet Coke man can get his shirt off, but also bringing plateaus and injuries to seasoned veterans.

What's more important is doing the right *type* of exercise.

To drop fat your focus shouldn't be on how many calories you can burn while working out. It should be on two things: Stimulating your lean tissue (muscle) and prompting calorie burning *after* your workout!

A workout is there to give instructions to our body. It's in between our workouts that our body is following those instructions and making changes.

As we've established, working out to burn calories is a false economy that will trap you on that hamster wheel. However, by working our muscles in the right way we can create what's called the afterburn effect, where you'll be burning calories long after the workout has ended.

Plus by stimulating your muscle you'll look shapely and more toned instead of thinner but still flabby, and you'll increase your day-to-day metabolism to boot.

Win-win!

Lean Living Rule #3: Working Out *Longer* Won't Improve Your Results

Seeing a pattern? When people don't see results because of number one, first they'll do more (number two), then they'll do it for longer. 20 minute workouts become 30 minutes. 30 becomes 45.

The results aren't in the duration though. Like I said, you need to hit 90 minutes before fat burning even *starts!* And how many hard-bodies that you stalk on Instagram do you think are working out for 2 hours a day? Almost none of them.

The results are in the intensity, and the longer you work for, the more the intensity gets diluted.

Or to put it another way, you can't sprint a marathon.

There's also other down sides for exercising for too long. Past 45 minutes, you start to produce more of the hormone cortisol in large amounts. Cortisol is a stress hormone responsible for depositing fat on your abdomen and weight retention, i.e. making it more difficult to lose weight and, just to kick you while you're down, sticking it on your belly!

Now, how big the actual impact all of this will have on your results in the world outside the science lab is hard to say, but when you consider you can get results that are just as good from much less, *and* have time left over to live your life, is spending hours working out every week actually worth it?

So look for ways to make your exercise *harder*, not longer. Increase the difficulty of the exercises you're doing. Increase the resistance. Lower your rest time. In *'Part 3: Get Up'* I'm going to lay out a bunch of workouts for you that you can take straight from the page.

Chapter 2

The Four Letter Success Killer

"Dieting is easy. It's like riding a bike. Except the bike is on fire. And the ground is on fire. And everything's on fire because you're in Hell."

– Unknown

Diet. If there's one thing that will stop you from getting lasting permanent results it's those four letters.

It's a sneaky little word, because it *almost* leads you down the right path. As we mentioned before, it actually does address the root cause: the food we eat. The problem, though, is the *way* it addresses it. It's like addressing a cold with paracetamol. It masks the symptoms for you so you can get on with your day, but the problem (the cold) is still there waiting to jump up and bite you on the arse once you stop taking it.

It's temporary. So temporary in fact two thirds of people who go on a diet not only gain back everything they lost, but gain back *more*!

Plus there's the negative connotations that come with the word. I surveyed people on my Facebook page and asked one simple question: What does the word "Diet" mean to you?

Here's a few of the replies:

- "Deprivation"

- "Depression"

- "Being hungry"

- "Feeling miserable"

- "Boring"

- "Restriction"

Seeing a pattern? This was my personal favourite:

- "A fight for something I'll never achieve."

Now THAT'S depressing!

When you go on a diet, you've basically already made the decision that you're going to fail. And like Henry Ford said, "Whether you think you can or you think you can't, you're right!"

What you think affects how you feel, and how you feel affects the actions you take. It's a knock-on effect. And if you look at what you're eating as deprivation, restriction, or any number of negative words you're fighting a losing battle.

Having that negative attitude when making food choices just causes emotional frustration, and ultimately overeating. You can even start to resent healthy foods and reach for the unhealthy choices for comfort or even as an internal rebellion!

If you just change the way you look at it, you can approach your eating with empowering thoughts instead.

Reframe it

Instead of focusing on what you *can't* eat or what you think you have to give up, think about all the things you *can* eat. Think about the new and exciting foods and recipes you can try.

Think about the positive results you'll get because of what you're eating. Think about your waistline tightening. Think about your hips shrinking. Think about slipping into that killer dress you used to absolutely rock, but now just push aside in your wardrobe in favour of the one that hides all your wobbly bits.

Think, "It's not that I *can't* eat that, I'm just making the healthier choice not to."

Can't is someone else dictating and restricting you. Choosing not to is empowerment.

Recently myself and my fiancée, Nic, were part of a conversation about being offered things by friends. Little things. That slice of cake because their daughter just turned two. That biscuit with your cuppa.

They'll say things like, *"Life's too short, just have the biscuit"*, or, *"It's all about balance"*.

Then Nic said something that completely summed up the situation:

"Life might be too short when it's that random one-off dessert in a flash restaurant on a special occasion. Less so when it's a packet of hobnobs being passed round the office every day!"

Exactly.

So remember, "It's not that I *can't* eat that, I'm just making the healthier choice not to."

Change Your Vocabulary

Stop using the word 'diet' and start using terms like, 'healthy lifestyle', because that's what it is. It's not a diet. It's a lifestyle.

There's another quote I love: "Athletes don't diet and exercise, they eat and train."

They're not dieting, they're just eating. Simple changes to the language you use when you speak and think can completely change your perception of what you're doing.

Relearn How to Eat

In psychology there are four stages of competence and each of them relates to how we eat. Understanding them will mean we never have to diet again:

- **Unconscious Incompetence:** In terms of your eating and nutrition, this is where most people are now. Our eating isn't mindful. We eat because we're hungry, because food was put in front of us, because somebody made a cup of tea, or because we happened to walk down the crisp aisle and remembered how much we like Frazzles. We don't pay any real attention to what we eat past maybe the odd fleeting, "A minute on the lips" joke with the lady behind the counter at Puffy Pastries.

- **Conscious Incompetence:** This is where we still have no idea what we're doing, but know the problem exists. So this time we'll make the joke, but inside we'll know maybe we shouldn't be buying our lunch at Puffy Pastries.

- **Conscious Competence:** This is where you'll be when you start applying the principles in this programme. You'll now know what to do and be applying the information, but you'll be very aware of it, and it will take thought and effort on your part. Like learning to drive a car. You have to concentrate on lifting your left foot at the same time as pushing your right down. You also know for sure now not to drive to Puffy Pastries.

- **Unconscious Competence:** This is where you don't need to think about what you're eating, you just do it. Like when you've been driving a while, your hands and feet move automatically so you can freely belt out that awesome 80s power ballad you pretend you don't like on the radio (and totally nail it... Obviously) and wave at the lady in Puffy Pastries while you drive past on the way to the gym.

How do you navigate your way through these 4 stages? Take the time to *re-learn* how to eat, then make it habit.

Be a bit neurotic about it early on if it helps. Set alarms to eat if you need to. Measure your portions. But whatever you do, don't half-arse it.

Stick to the plan for just 21 days, which is enough time to start forming new habits so you never have to put any real thought into eating again.

And whatever you do, I want you to promise me one thing.

Never go on a diet again.

Chapter 3

The Five Ps

"Give me six hours to chop down a tree and I will spend the first four sharpening the axe."

– Abraham Lincoln

When I was a wee young lad, I was in the cub scouts. Every week I'd tighten my woggle, pull down my cap, and stand in a cold hall in my little grey shorts with 15 or so other young boys reciting an oath to a flag.

When the time came, I didn't get to go to big-boy scouts because I had to make the choice of either going to proper scouts or having drum lessons. I wasn't allowed both... Music lessons aren't cheap you know!

At the time though, Bear Grylls was barely a teenager, and I wanted to be like Animal from the Muppets. True, I was about 10 or something, but if I'm honest, given the choice again today, I'd probably still choose to emulate that crazy puppet!

There was a great lesson I learned in the cubs though, and that's to be prepared. Although they summed it up in two words, I also like this saying — What I call the 5 Ps (or 6 Ps as I usually tell it, but I'm going to keep this book PG rated!):

Proper Planning Prevents Poor Performance.

Now, I'm not one for wishy washy management speak. We won't be doing any 'blue sky thinking' or 'nailing any jellies to the wall' in here. But planning and preparing what you're going to eat can quite literally be the difference between massive rip-roaring success and utter dismal failure.

See, planning your week in advance doesn't take long, especially after you're a couple of weeks into your programme. Most people eat the same breakfast and the same lunch every day, and the only real variance is their dinner. Even if you prefer your eating to be much more diverse over the week, you could easily repeat that same week over and over just adjusting for events, or schedule deviations you know are coming.

Preparation doesn't take long either. It doesn't take any longer to cook six portions of a meal than it does to cook one, and now you have five meals in your fridge for the coming week. And even if you scaled that down to just cooking one extra portion at dinner time, that's lunch for the next day done. No thinking about it in the morning, no getting it ready, just taking it out of the fridge, done.

Being prepared takes away two huge hurdles – decision making and time.

Did you know Facebook CEO Mark Zuckerberg reportedly wears the same outfit every day? Weird, right? Or is it actually genius?

When you're the owner of the biggest social media network in the world, you have to make a lot of decisions. Even if you're a prodigy like Zuckerberg you suffer from a condition called *decision fatigue.*

Psychologist Roy F. Baumeister said, "Making decisions uses the very same willpower that you use to say no to doughnuts, drugs, or illicit sex"

If you already know what you're having for lunch tomorrow, there's no danger of being faced with so many options that you just go 'screw it' and make some toast. Admit it, it happens more than you'd like! Also without that need to even look at options, there's no room for temptation.

And all it takes is setting aside half an hour or so once or twice per week.

Here's how to make planning and preparing a piece of, well, cake!

Gather Some Go-to Meals

Start by making a master list of your favourite meals that fit the plan. It doesn't need to be extensive either, just 5-10 favourites you can rotate in will be enough to generate several weeks of meal plans. Knock out a list of 10-15 and you'll be covered for the next several months! Especially if you're like most people and tend to eat the same breakfast and same lunch most days of the week.

When you have your list, store it however works best for you. In your phone, in a notebook, on a pin-board, in a spreadsheet. Whatever you identify with and can access quickly. Then when it comes to writing your meal plans, you can just dip in, choose a meal, and essentially just fill in the gaps!

Good Eating Starts with Good Shopping

There's a very simple principle: If you don't buy it, you can't eat it. So always shop from a list, and never shop hungry!

When you're hungry, everything looks tempting and food just seems to leap into your trolley with no outside help! "Oh look, profiteroles are two for one. That's a bargain. I'd best take four just to make sure."

"Hey look, they have scabby donkey on sale..."

Enter with a full belly and a plan, and only go down the aisles you need.

If you want extra pro-points, do your shopping online. This has a tonne of advantages:

- The website will save your shopping list. Just do it once, and although you may have to make a few minor adjustments, then you can basically just click and go. Although as loyalty cards like to track what you've bought in the past you might want to quickly go through the "Favourites" and get rid of the cheeky packet of biscuits you bought six weeks ago.

- There's no temptation anymore! All the come-hither smells from the food counters, or the checkouts lined with chocolates. It's all just sterile photos of food packets.

- You, of course, don't lose an hour of your day fighting traffic just to schlep up and down artificially lit aisles. That hour could be spent working out or preparing your food plan or meals for the week.

Batch Process

As I mentioned earlier, it doesn't take any longer to cook six servings of a meal than it does to cook one, so when you're cooking your dinner one day, cook up several servings and chuck the ones you're not eating in Tupperware.

Or just set aside half an hour to an hour to cook up a bunch of your go-to meals at a set time in the week.

There's a bit of an in-joke in the fitness world where Sunday is International Meal Prep day. It's the day fit people the world over get out a stack of Tupperware and their big saucepan, then just spend 30-60 minutes or so diligently cooking up meals for the coming week. They then spend the rest of the week stroking their abs while doing squats and updating their Instagram account with all the time they saved.

OK, so I may have made that last bit up, and you don't necessarily have to join this ritual, but even if you scaled it down to overcooking a few times per week, think how much time, effort, and energy you'll save during the week.

Make a note of which meals you can batch cook and put in the fridge. Which meals will last a few days there? Which ones could you freeze for even longer periods?

Think about your upcoming schedule and where you're going to be. Which meals are portable? Which ones do you need a microwave for? Which ones could you eat straight out of the tub in your car if you had to?

Then all you need to do is plug-and-play. Insert the relevant meal into the relevant part of your day.

Meal prepping doesn't need to be difficult or complicated any more than meal planning does. And given that you're reading this book you're busy enough that you probably already do some degree of meal planning for you and your family any way, whether you realise it or not! What those one to two hours a week will do for you though is free up several times those hours for you, and not only automate your body transformation, but automate a large part of your life too! And that makes room for more of the fun stuff in life!

Chapter 4

Afterburn:
Burn Fat
While You Sleep

"Exercise would be so much more rewarding if calories screamed while you burned them."

– Unknown

I remember once many years ago watching a great video that properly illustrated the problem. In the video were two guys. One was on a treadmill, and the other had a slice of pizza. Just one large slice, this wasn't man vs food or anything, but that slice of pizza was about 500-600 calories.

The task at hand was straight forward. The guy on the treadmill was going to run for the same amount of time it took the other guy to eat his pizza slice.

So one was burning calories, the other ingesting them.

So off they went. One guy started chowing down on the pizza – Not fast, but not slow either, and the other guy went for it on the treadmill. This was proper hell for leather too! He was sprinting like Wile E. Coyote had laced Road Runner's bird seed with speed.

It took the one guy less than 2 minutes to get through the 500-odd calorie slice of pizza. On the other hand, by sprinting for 2 minutes, the runner had burned around 33 calories.

So the point was pretty obvious! You can take in 500 odd calories quicker than a Taylor Swift break-up, but to burn that off, that 1 single slice of pizza, you would have to sprint for over half an hour. (And yes, it's impossible to sprint for 30 minutes, but you get the point!)

In short, trying to burn off what you eat through exercise is a false economy. Remember Lean Living Rule #1? Unless you're an extreme endurance athlete, you're never going to burn enough calories during exercise to even make a dent.

However, there is a way to use exercise to keep on burning long after you've stepped off the treadmill – real or metaphorical – and that's using a concept we call "Afterburn".

The technical name for this is Excess Post-Exercise Oxygen Consumption (EPOC), and what we're referring to is how many calories you burn after the exercise as a result of the exercise. I.e. how long and how much after you step out of the gym you're still burning calories for.

Now, different types of exercise will raise your metabolism by different amounts for different lengths of time.

Doing long, steady cardio, for example, will raise it a little bit for a few hours. Traditional strength (resistance/weight) training will raise it a bit more and for longer

And then there's a type of training called Metabolic Resistance Training.

This has been shown to raise your metabolism for as much as 18 hours after stepping out of the gym!

In some cases this has continued for 24, or even 48 hours, but even in a worst case scenario, 18 hours is a LONG time to be burning extra calories! And this will all be happening in the background – even while you sleep!

Oh, and as a bonus, as well as increasing your muscle strength and tone, it's also been shown to improve your cardio fitness as much as traditional steady-state cardio with workouts that are completed in a fraction of the time.

There's no downside here!

So how do we do that? Well, Metabolic Resistance Training is a combination of both strength training and cardio training. So whereas you'd traditionally hit the weights for, say, 45-60 minutes, then afterwards (or separately to) you'd do your cardio, we're going to use a technique that combines the two into one short but intense workout.

When we do that, a synergistic effect happens so the results you get are *better* than the sum of the parts. We'll talk more about synergism in the next chapter with what I call "Success Stacking".

Here's how it works: You'll work in short bursts of 2-4 minutes performing strength based exercises, then rest for a minute or two, then go again, keeping this up for anything from 10-30 minutes.

By using the strength based exercises that we know create the biggest stimulus and demand the most out of our body, then combining that with the short rest times, we create a big demand on our cardiovascular system too.

As a result, for the next 18 or so hours, your body is still going through its recovery and regeneration, followed by the overcompensation (getting fitter and stronger) phase, and to fuel that, it needs extra calories.

Or to put it more simply, you've created a stimulus, and now you're sitting back while your body capitalises on it – even when you're watching Corrie!

Now, understand this, the other thing that pizza video taught us was that even when you're burning calories for hours, if you rely just on exercise, you'll still need plenty of hours to so much as break even! So you'll still need to make sure you're following a targeted fat burning nutrition plan...

...But put the two together, and the results can be spectacular.

Chapter 5

Success Stacking: Putting It All Together

"Great things are done by a series of small things brought together."

– Vincent Van Gogh

The secret to this programme's effectiveness is not in the parts, but the stacking of those parts. We're taking lots of little things which, on their own will edge you a little way forward but when stacked together though something magical happens — Synergism.

Not just a sexy word, synergism means that when you stack the right things together, they work so beautifully in cooperation that the result is greater than the sum of its parts.

A Hache Steak tastes great on its own, but add onions and a slice of cheese, and it takes the flavour to new levels. Throw in some lettuce and tomato and this basic steak is becoming something special. Garnish with peppercorn sauce and rest it on a lightly toasted bun and suddenly Heaven's knocking on your door asking to come to dinner!

Mmmmmm... Sorry, what were we talking about?

It creates a snowball effect. You start with basics, then layer up with smaller things, and add garnish on the top, and by doing so you create a synergistic effect.

It's what I call 'Success Stacking' and it works like this:

- **OK:** Working out will burn some calories during that workout and get you a little success.

- **AWESOME:** Working out in the right way (Metabolic Resistance Training) will...

  o Create an 'afterburn' effect that burns calories for hours afterwards and into the next day.

  o Build body-toning and shaping muscle that can burn 50+ calories per pound of bodyweight.

- **OK:** Dieting or controlling your calories will create an energy deficit, letting you lose some weight (both fat and muscle), but ultimately lowering your metabolism, reducing how many calories you burn every day.

- **AWESOME:** Eating a simple balanced plan of smaller, regular meals, that's designed to fuel your muscles while forcing your body to use stored fat as energy will...

  o Pushup your metabolism several times per day by providing a predictable, frequent nutritional intake.

  o Allow your body to let go of the fat because it knows there's always nutrition around the corner so has no need to store it

- o   Provide all the building blocks for that new slimming, body-shaping, calorie-burning muscle.

You see how these things start to interact and add up?

Now let's stack those two awesome things together. Suddenly the parts are becoming bigger than themselves.

- Our Metabolic Resistance workouts are now pushing our metabolism up for hours after we've walked out of the gym.

- Every time we eat, we spike our metabolism, so by eating smaller, more frequent meals we're pushing it up several times per day.

- By eating the right balance of proteins, carbohydrates, and fat, we're now creating new lean, toned muscle which pushes our metabolism up 24/7.

We've now turned you into a fat-burning machine! But let's not stop there...

On top of that let's add in some other things that we can do every day like drinking ice-cold water to push our metabolism up a little bit more, taking a nightly walk with your water bottle after dinner, or any number of little things I've listed in the 'Ramp It Up' chapter for you later on.

Not only do they add up fast but little things are easier to manage and easier to work into your lifestyle.

Little changes are easy to make and much easier to maintain.

But most of all, little things build big things. One brick won't do much on its own. Stack enough of them though and you have the Great Wall of China.

One Step at a Time

We know that all these little things add up, but very few people can just start implementing them all at once. It takes time... Especially to form new lasting habits that make this stuff run on auto-pilot!

In fact the studies show transforming one new habit at a time gives you an 80% chance of being successful. Add one more habit and your success rate drops to 20%.

But the fact is, you don't need to switch it all on overnight. How do you do it?

Pick one and focus on it and it alone for 3-7 days.

For example, one of my clients never ate breakfast because, she thought, she never had time. She did however have time to drink her tea in the morning. She's British after-all!

So I gave her a smoothie recipe and now she drinks that instead.

Great! Breakfast sorted. Tick it off the list.

Then it was struggling to eat throughout the day because, again, she didn't have time to prepare meals for herself. So I gave her the homework of overcooking at dinner time and storing up the portions for the next few days.

That's it. One thing. She's nailed the breakfast thing, now time to focus on something else.

If you just focused on one thing each week, 6 weeks down the line you've made big changes. There's 52 weeks in a year. Change just one thing per week and this time next year you won't even recognise yourself.

Chapter 6

Ready, Fire, Aim

"Just do it."

– Nike

I watched a great video recently which, although wasn't about fitness, made a really good point.

When you purchase something, it's like scratching an itch.

So for example, if you have 20, 30, 40, whatever pounds to lose, taking that step by buying a manual or joining a weight loss programme will immediately make you feel better about it. You haven't fixed the situation, but you've taken the first step to doing that.

You've scratched the itch.

When you bought this book, you scratched the itch.

But what happens after that? You need to follow through. When you scratched that itch, you made a commitment to yourself.

So when that mood has left you, when that itch has been tended to, you still need to put the effort in, even if you don't feel like it.

That's what separates the successes from the failures. Not effort, not action, but CONSISTENT effort and action.

"A successful life is the sum total of several successful years. A successful year is the sum total of 12 successful months. A successful month is the sum total of 4-5 successful weeks. A successful week is the sum total of 7 successful days. A successful day is the sum total of 24 successful hours."

That quote is from the late Bob Safford. Back in 2011, I had the great pleasure of being able to learn directly from Mr Safford. He was insightful, witty, made his first million by age 28, and had coached and mentored thousands of people on how to do the same.

And yes, I did say made his first million by age 28! And I can tell you, the things highly successful people in all areas have in common, including money making or body transformation, is no coincidence.

You see everything we do is habitual. It's routine. The way we get ready in the morning right down to the way we eat.

Tony Schwartz and James E. Loehr talk about this a lot in their book, "The Power of Full Engagement".

Psychologists reckon it takes around 21 days to change a habit. That means we need to consciously do something for around 3 weeks before it becomes automatic. So if you're starting a new fitness plan, allow yourself to be a bit "neurotic" about it in the early stages. Set alarms to remind you when to eat. Plan meticulously and schedule your workouts.

Yes, it's hard work at first, and yes it's a pain in the arse, but nothing worth doing is easy. The first 21 days is where you tend to separate the people who are serious from everyone else.

If you are serious, after that first 21 days it becomes much easier. Almost automatic. Like cleaning your teeth!

So if you want to not only be successful, but put that success on autopilot, you need to follow 3 steps:

Step 1 — Scratch the itch: You bought this book and have got this far. You can tick this one off!

Step 2 — Take action: Learning what to do isn't enough. Knowing the steps you have to take isn't enough. You have to take action. You don't even have to get it right! Just start taking forward steps, gather momentum and make corrections as you go.

Step 3 — Lather, rinse, repeat: Once you're taking those forward steps, repeat them. Repetition forms new habits, and new habits are the key to more effortless results.

Right now though, I don't want you to wait until everything's perfect. I don't want you to spend the next fortnight planning every meal you're going to eat, or every workout you're going to do. As soon as you've put this book down, I just want you to get started.

Inspiration
Kelie Hoadley

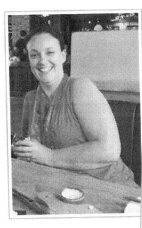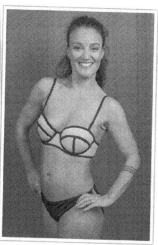

Sitting here, typing this, I can't quite believe what I've lost; 37 lbs, several inches and the wish to be invisible. More importantly I can't believe what I've gained; strength – of all kinds – a fitness level that allows me to pull off my very best crazy lady dance moves without collapsing and a body that I genuinely never thought I'd see again.

There were several cringe moments that started me on the path back to fitness, but my before photo sums it up in one shot really, I was out with my Mum and beautiful daughter, eating Tapas to celebrate her turning 8 months old and I thought I wasn't looking too bad that day – I'd made an effort for once, put on a colourful top and scarf and had even found some clean leggings. But looking at the photo I realised not only was I bigger than I'd thought, but I didn't put makeup on anymore and I didn't know how long my hair was because it only ever got washed and jammed into a Mum-bun.

I was raising two children and had great hopes of teaching them (amongst other things!) that women are to be treasured, respected and valued whatever they look like and here I was hiding in plain sight because I didn't like the way I looked. I was mourning my pre-baby body, punishing myself for changing while creating these glorious creatures and I needed to stop.

After a hideous 14 days doing a juice detox cleanse (read: two week long starvation because those things are disgusting) I found Anthony and a home based workout programme, and without knowing it then, changed my life. I did the workouts at home, much to the bemusement of the kids, and was startled to find that although most of what I was eating was good, I was possibly eating three people's worth. I was also very good at not eating anything during the day and then having a huge pasta dinner with a pile of cheese. The novelty of three meals a day plus two snacks felt very indulgent for a while!

I was really pleased with the results and ended up doing two 6 week programmes back to back. Christmas came and I gave myself a couple of weeks off and signed up for his 28 day challenge in January to undo the festive damage and ramp things up a bit. That involved doing the classes at his studio which terrified me, images of being surrounded by Goddesses' planking and leaping about gracefully while I thundered and panted like a warthog had me shaking that first morning. But the people, and the instructor were lovely, there were options through all of the exercises so I could do what worked for me without feeling like a failure and I left on a real high.

My determination was set; I followed that eating plan to the letter, scraped ice off the car at 5:30am three times a week to get to the studio and lost 12 lbs in those 28 days. I not only felt very much part of the team but as if I was getting a sense of self back. Doing something for myself and getting genuine results. It was the happiest I'd been for ages!

I was hooked, continued with the classes and eating plan and within a year I'd completed a 'bikini body' challenge which ended with a bikini clad photo shoot, something which I would have avoided at any cost less than 12 months previously.

I recently got married was lucky enough to have a honeymoon on a beach. I felt confident in my skin on the day and on the holiday which was wonderful, but what has surprised me is the number of people who've asked if I'm going to stop doing my "silly gym thing" now that the wedding is over. I totally understand that getting up at 5:15am in order to be bossed about by super humans doesn't appeal to everyone but this was never about getting into a particular dress or looking good for one holiday.

As one of the many who have pretty much battled against my own body for most of my life, through the savages of Anorexia in my teenage years and various relapses in times of stress since, I'm never quite free of the darkness that threatens to consume again every time life gets out of control.

This is what I do for myself now, this is my time; time without children, without a million demands, without being constantly interrupted to find something, provide something, do something. This is my control.

I cope better with life now and with the kids, my body is healthy and strong and that is reflected in all the other parts of me. My jeans no longer fit, in a good way, and my hair and makeup are done more often than not. Anthony is awesome, he makes us remember that we are too.

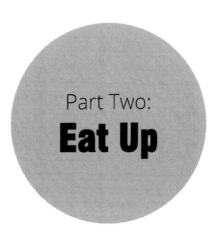

Part Two:
Eat Up

Chapter 7

Creating Your New Normal

"The food you eat can be either the safest and most powerful form of medicine or the slowest form of poison."

– Ann Wigmore

As we talked about earlier, if you want to lose a significant amount of body fat, there's one part of your lifestyle that will need looking at above everything else, and that's what you eat. No-one is overweight purely because they don't do enough exercise.

Or to put it another way, it's not what you put your body through, it's what you put through your body.

But true to eating well and acts of war alike, before we can design an effective eating plan, we must know our enemy: Body fat.

The way we eat shouldn't just be to lose weight. Losing weight is easy: Eat fewer calories than you expend... And don't get me wrong, that is incredibly important (which I'll come back to later).

But we don't just want to lose *weight*. Just losing *weight* is a one-way ticket to looking thin and flabby. True, we do want to lose the wobbly stuff, said Captain Obvious, and we do do that by eating a little bit less... But we *also* need to nourish our muscle so we can be lean and shapely, *not* thin and flabby!

Let's be honest... If we were all firm and toned, we wouldn't give a monkeys how much we weighed!

So, let's go back to the beginning. What is body fat? Why do we have it?

Body fat, in the simplest terms, is just stored energy waiting to be used. Every day we ingest a certain number of calories, some of which are used to perform our daily tasks, and the excess is stored for a later date on our hips, or our stomach... Well anywhere really!

Once we have stored body fat, we then need to eat fewer calories than we use for our daily activities to tap into this stored energy source.

Now, read that last sentence again!

Everyone knows this bit, right? It's why when we need to lose fat everyone gets themselves stuck on that hamster wheel we talked about right at the beginning!

But these are complicated times we live in, and with instant access to more and more information, this simple universal truth is just flat-out ignored by a lot of diets.

It's just not sexy enough to keep our attention.

So instead they focus on dropping carbs, dropping fat, eating carbs only in the evening, or combining different nutrients at different times of the day... And sometimes they succeed too. *But when they do it's because 9 times out of 10 that person is eating less than their daily needs as a result.*

The Twinkie Diet

With all those bat-crap crazy ideas that are coming out of the diet industry right now, it's easy to think that maybe we've all just forgotten about the basic energy-in vs. energy-out equation. But one guy selflessly pulled on his lab coat and performed another bat-crap crazy idea to actually prove it!

That guy was Mark Haub who's a professor of human nutrition at Kansas State University. For 10 weeks, he set out to eat a diet made up mostly of Twinkies while keeping his calorie intake under his maintenance to lose weight.

If you don't know what a Twinkie is, it's a (according to the packet) *"Golden Sponge Cake with Creamy Filling."* It's also the only thing, other than cockroaches, they reckon will survive a nuclear holocaust.

So, in the interests of science, over those 10 weeks, he selflessly took a bullet for us all and made this weirdly indestructible spongy creaminess around two-thirds of his diet, with some other junk food thrown in for good measure.

What a hero.

The other third was still healthy, but here's the important bit: Despite the reliance on junk food, in 10 weeks he lost 27 pounds.

That's nearly two stone!

Now, don't get me wrong, a (probably large!) percentage of that loss would have been the lean stuff, and the experiment wasn't put forward as an advert for a long-term healthy lifestyle (or even a short-term weight-loss plan!), but what it proved was that when you strip away the over-complication and the pseudoscience, take in less than you expend and you'll lose weight.

We're not looking for a short-term plaster over the problem though, we need to focus on not only ridding our body of our soft, squidgy outer coating, but instilling new healthy, energising habits we can sustain for a lifetime. And in my experience, the key to doing this is to KISS.

"Keep It Super Simple!"

We're not going to focus on overly complicated food combining, or even calorie or point counting. Instead we're going to focus on a simple balance of nutrients over a wide range of foods, and I'm even going to show you how to get the right portion size every time, wherever, whenever.

Back in "Set Up" we talked about how your eating plan *shouldn't* make you feel. Deprived. Weak. Starving.

It should make you feel strong. Empowered even.

It should be simple, yet diverse. Straight-forward yet flexible.

I'm going to show you how to stop dieting and start living!

Chapter 8

Super Simple
Eating

*"Never eat ingredients you can't pronounce. Except quinoa.
You should eat quinoa."*

– Unknown

So now we understand that when it comes down to it, when you strip
away the over-complication, the science and the pseudoscience,
whichever source they come from calories are just fuel for our engines.
But different types of fuel are utilised in the body in different ways. By
balancing them in optimum amounts, we can significantly increase the
effects of what we're pumping in.

In the interests of KISS, to get a good balance we can organise our foods
into five basic categories:

Proteins, Fats, Starches, Fruits, and Vegetables.

The last three are all carbohydrates, and there's a reason I've split them
into three different categories.

Carbohydrates

Over the past decade or so, carbohydrates – or "Carbs" if you're down with the kids – have been demonised more than wearing socks with sandals. They've been accused of doing everything from layering fat on your body to sleeping with your significant other behind your back.

Probably.

You may have even seen complicated carb timing techniques, only being able to eat them on certain days of the week, before or after a workout, or before 6, 7, 8, or whatever in the evening.

But carbohydrates are just misunderstood.

Now, first off, don't get me wrong, if you're going that extra mile for a photo shoot or thinking of stepping on stage in a sparkly bikini and heels, then absolutely, carbohydrates can be timed and cycled to get you in that extraordinary shape. But if that's NOT your goal, and you just want to maintain a year-round hot-bod, then you don't need to complicate your life like that. I'm sure you have enough things going on to worry about without having to check your watch before eating an apple.

Carbs are the catalyst to the fat burning process. The fire lighters. And they also provide you with the energy you need to power through and recover from your workouts.

There are two basic types of carbs that you need to know about.

Simple carbs like those found in sweets and chocolate burn very quickly and give you a swift energy burst. Complex carbs such as rice and pasta (starches) provide a more drawn out energy supply with fewer energy dips and spikes.

For maximum fat burning, we want to get most of our carbs from the complex side of the family.

Protein

Ask most people, and when they think of protein, they'll think muscle. And rightly so. One fifth of your muscle tissue is protein so we do need to make sure we're getting enough to guarantee the right result.

We don't need to overload on protein, but it's important to make sure you're eating some with almost every meal.

One gram of protein provides around four calories, and although calories are our body's fuel, calories from protein are not the body's first choice as an energy source. In fact, it's the last. Only when the body is depleted of carbohydrates and fat will it use protein for energy.

They might not be great for energy, but protein calories come with a lot of handy little benefits, and one in particular is where it really comes into its own – What's called the thermic effect!

As well as supplying calories, all nutrients require a certain amount of calories to be digested, so there's a bit of an offset going on. Out of protein, carbs, and fats, protein has the highest thermic effect at 30%.

So to put this into perspective, for every 100 calories of protein you eat, you'll burn around 30 of them digesting and processing it. Remember when we talked about those little things that add up?

It's also the nutrient most responsible for making us feel fuller. So whichever way you slice it, upping our protein a bit is a big win all round!

Fat

Despite all the anti-fat propaganda you hear, some fats are actually very good for us, and in appropriate amounts can help reduce cholesterol and protect against heart disease.

Fats like that found in coconut oil, nuts and nut butters, avocado, and oily fish shouldn't be ignored. Instead they should be enthusiastically embraced in the same way that one over-affectionate auntie always leaves lipstick on your face at the family Christmas party.

It's worth remembering though that fats pack a weighty 9 calories per gram. That's more than double what's supplied by the same weight of carbs or protein, so we don't need to overload on them to get the right effect.

Grazing

To keep the fat burners locked in fifth gear all through the day, you should aim to eat smaller meals more often rather than the standard three big meals per day. This can be done in a number of ways, but one way I've found to work consistently is simply to scale down your usual main meals and then add small snacks in between.

By eating like this you never leave your body hungry. If you were to eat only 3 times per day, the gaps between these meals would be pretty lengthy! If done regularly, this can be perceived by our body as potential future starvation, and your body's defence against this is to create energy stores. I.e. body fat.

Apart from the obvious reasons why we don't want to store body fat, there is also the fact that if these nutrients are being stored up for later bouts of "starvation", they are not being given to our muscles so they can repair and build after a workout.

Alcohol

OK, you knew it was coming! The elephant in the room. The dreaded A-word.

We all know alcohol and stripping body-fat don't mix very well, and don't shoot the messenger here, but if you're a 'couple of glasses of wine a night to unwind' kinda gal, you're going to need to rethink your drinking habits a bit if you're really serious about ditching that wobbly stuff.

Now, I'm not saying you need to give it up because you don't, we just need to get properly educated about the subject so we can get it in without shooting ourselves in the foot with a rocket launcher.

Here's some quick and dirty alcohol facts:

- 1 small glass of wine (pub measure) has around 100-150 calories. 1 pint of beer has around 150-200 calories. What's worse though is that those calories have no real nutritional value, so they're what we call "empty" calories.

- Alcohol is a preferred source of energy to body fat and needs to be burned first. As long as there's alcohol in your system, your body isn't burning fat.

- Alcohol suppresses the hormones in your body responsible for burning fat and building the lean stuff for up to 48 hours after you've necked your last 'Sex on the beach'.

That means over the course of an evening, you can easily rack up a large chunk of your daily calories with these empty calories. And of course, that's not including what you've already eaten that day, and what you'll eat during and after (including that kebab you'll probably forget you had on the way home).

Then, to add insult to injury, on top of having all those extra calories to burn before your body even thinks about shifting fat out of your system, its ability to do so is impaired for the next day or two.

The key to having your booze and drinking it too is not to do it little and often, and it's not to binge either. It's to find the happy medium.

For long term fat loss, a glass of wine two or three times per week probably won't hurt you (pub measures – put the pint glass down!).

Three or four glasses of wine one night per week probably won't hurt you either.

Do both of those on any given week, and you'll probably be going nowhere.

If you have an event coming up though, or you're really serious and you just want to drop the fat as quickly as your body will allow, then the best option is to drop the alcohol altogether for a four to six week block, so your body can really take some giant leaps forward, and then finding that happy medium if you still find you fancy a glass every now and then.

Chapter 9

Super Simple Portions

"For many years, my formula has been to love yourself, move your body and to watch portion size. But the No. 1 thing is to love and value yourself, no matter what you've been through."

– Richard Simmons

When Is Healthy Eating Not Eating Healthily?

Often when people are standing in front of me for the first time, they'll tell me they eat healthily. When I ask them what they eat they'll reel off a typical day's food that's cleaner than a cat's nipples... But they still have 10, 20, 30 or more pounds they want to lose.

Now, your first instinct is probably that they're not being completely honest about what they're eating, and a lot of times you'd be right, but you *can* eat incredibly healthily and still perpetually gain weight down to one simple reason: Portion size.

As we discussed before, you can eat an awful diet that you'd only think was healthy if you'd been hit around the head a few times with a Big Mac. But if you obey the simple rule that you eat slightly less calories than you expend, you'll still lose weight.

Well the same happens in reverse.

Eat too much of a good thing and you create a calorie surplus, and those calories still need to go somewhere. Like it or not, that somewhere's most likely going to be your bum, thighs, and belly!

And you have to ask yourself, if your healthy diet is perpetually causing you to gain weight, is it still healthy?

I'm going to hang right off the end of this limb here and say, "Not so much".

In probably 9 cases out of 10, the very first thing that needs addressing for anyone who has weight to lose is portion size.

The biggest problem with portion size is that, because we generally have no idea what an appropriate portion size is, we use our plates and bowls as measuring devices. We fill up our dinner plates. We pour things into bowls until they reach the top. And before we know it those calories have shot up faster than Jeremy Clarkson's blood pressure.

But on the other hand, we don't wander around with kitchen scales or measuring cups in our pockets. We don't need to though. We can get the portion size right wherever, whenever using that other thing we wander around with in our pockets... No, not your phone — Your hand.

In the beginning of Chapter 8 we broke everything you eat down into 5 food groups. Here's how to use your hand to get the portion size right every time:

Protein and Starches: Size of the palm of your hand

Vegetables: Size of your closed fist

Fruits: Should fit in your cupped hand

Fats: Size of your thumb

Simple, right? If you eat a protein food like chicken or fish, or if you eat a starchy carb like pasta, potatoes, or rice, it should be the same size as the palm of your hand. If you're serving up your veggies, the portion should be the size of your fist, and so on.

And by the way, your starches should be measured *after* cooking!

Your Full Day

Although how many portions you eat over the course of the day will take a little bit of trial and error, I've found most women will do well by starting here:

- 4-5 servings of Protein and the same of Starches

- 4-6 servings of Vegetables

- 2-3 servings of Fruits and the same of Fat

Fat dropping off comfortably? Great. Don't change a thing.

If it's hanging on like Debbie Harry on the phone, trim a bit from the top of your portion size. And I can't emphasise this enough, but keep it simple.

Micro-management

If you like to weigh, measure, and track numbers, particularly early on, that's not necessarily a bad way to be. Although it can seem a bit anal, what it will show you is what a portion size *should* look like, and exactly how much you should be eating daily, and if you're used to overeating, it can be a bit of a shock!

A good shock.

If this is you, I'd recommend grabbing a good set of digital kitchen scales and some cup and spoon measures. Here's how your portion sizes will break down now:

Protein and Starches: ½-⅔ Cup or 80-100g or 3-3 ½oz

Vegetables: 1 Cup

Fruits: ½ Cup or 1 piece

Fats: 1 Teaspoon

Tracking your calories for a week or two will also help you get used to how you can balance those serving sizes. Back in the day, we used to do this with a pocket-sized calorie counter — like those little dictionaries we used to carry around at school, but filled with foods — and a pen and paper. These days though, there's a whole bunch of apps you can download that will track everything from calories, to nutrients, to water. Some of them will even let you scan the packet's barcode to find something super-quick!

Try to keep between 1,200 and 1,500 calories to trim the wobbly stuff, aiming for around 30-40% protein, 30-40% carbohydrates, and 20-30% fat, and nearer 2,000 calories when you're maintaining your current shape.

What to Eat

It's great knowing your portion sizes, but it also helps knowing what foods are best suited to getting you to your goal.

Now, take note of that sentence. Not what foods are good and what foods are bad, because foods should be looked at in the context of your whole day. As we said before, the odd chocolate digestive isn't going to hurt your progress. Two chocolate digestives every day with your cup of tea probably will.

So what I've done is list what I would consider to be the *best* choices when deciding what to put in your mouth. Focus the majority of your eating around these foods, and you won't go far wrong.

Proteins

- Chicken breast
- Turkey breast
- Top round steak
- Top sirloin steak
- Lean beef mince (5% fat or less)
- Lean ham
- Haddock
- Cod
- Tuna
- Trout
- Lobster
- Shrimp
- Prawns
- Tofu
- Quorn
- Egg whites (limit yolks to 1-2 per day)
- Low-fat cottage cheese
- Low-fat soft cheese or quark

Carbohydrates

- Carbohydrates
- Pasta
- Rice
- Oats
- Baked potato
- Sweet potato
- Squash
- Pumpkin
- Barley
- Beans
- Kidney beans
- Lentils
- Chick peas
- Sweetcorn
- Corn
- Low-fat yoghurt
- Skimmed milk
- Wholemeal bread
- High-fibre cereal

Fruits

- Apples
- Apricots
- Bananas
- Blackberries
- Blueberries
- Cherries
- Clementines
- Dates
- Figs
- Grapefruit
- Melons

Vegetables

- Artichoke
- Asparagus
- Bean sprouts
- Beetroot
- Broccoli
- Brussels sprouts
- Cabbage
- Carrots
- Cauliflower
- Courgette
- Greens

- Kiwis
- Mangos
- Nectarines
- Oranges
- Papayas
- Peaches
- Pears
- Pineapples
- Plums
- Raspberries
- Strawberries
- Tangerines
- Watermelon

- Leeks
- Mushrooms
- Onion
- Peas
- Peppers
- Sauerkraut
- Beans (spring, green, yellow)
- Tomato
- Turnips

Fats

Good Fats:
- Unsalted nuts
- Extra virgin oil
- Nut oils
- Vegetable oils
- Sunflower oils
- Corn oils
- Coconut oil
- Oily fish (such as mackerel, salmon, and sardines)

Fats to eat sparingly:
- Fatty meats
- Whole milk
- Full fat cheese
- Oils that have been treated to make them semi-solid (such as margarines)

Chapter 10

Super Simple Hydration

"When you pour water in a cup, it becomes the cup. When you pour water in a bottle, it becomes the bottle. When you pour water in a teapot, it becomes the teapot. Water can drip and it can crash. Become like water my friend."

– Bruce Lee

One often neglected, yet ridiculously important part of the weight loss puzzle is drinking enough water. Our bodies, by weight, are made up of around 60% water. That's more than half! Yet time and time again, we just don't drink as much water as we should.

Oh, and before we go too much further, prosecco and tea don't count as water. I know. Sometimes life can really punch you in the jubblies.

But practically every function performed by the body requires water, some more important than others. The brain and heart, both pretty vital organs I reckon, can't function without a certain minimum amount of water present.

Here are a few other reasons we need water:

- It acts as a coolant by regulating the body's temperature, and removing excess heat through sweat.

- It acts as a lubricant to the joints and between internal organs.

- It acts as a solvent to water soluble vitamins.

- Skeletal muscles are made up of as much as 71% water.

- It helps keep skin clear and healthy.

- It aids digestion of food in the stomach and the digestive tract.

- It aids flushing the body of waste materials.

All good reasons why drinking water is good for you, but here's a few things that can happen when we don't:

- Headaches

- Lethargy, weakness

- Muscle cramps

- Dark yellow urine

- Dizziness

- Poor skin tone

We can probably tick at least half of these boxes off on any given day, right?

We put it down to stress or a hard day's work, when really we're just walking around in a state of partial dehydration.

But avoiding blackheads is just the tip of the watery iceberg. Apart from all the above, you need to make sure your kidneys are supplied with enough water, or you could be unwittingly slamming the brakes on your fat loss.

See, your kidneys are pretty needy. They're like that teenager who thinks they're independent, but really if they lost the Wi-Fi password, they wouldn't last the week.

They need a lot of water to function, but if they are not getting enough, they rely on the liver for help.

The liver has a lot on its plate already though, and one of its jobs is to get stored fat up off its arse so it can be useful and we can use it as energy. If the liver is helping the kidneys do their job, it's not concentrating on its own, indirectly compromising your fat loss.

Another, more cosmetic side effect of not drinking enough water is water retention.

You know those days your hormones are jumping around like a spider on a hot-plate? You feel puffy and soft. Bloated even. And every time you look in the mirror you feel like your usual reflection has jetted off to a hot country and left the Michelin Man behind to stand in for it.

Well if the body is not getting enough water, it will hold on to all the water it does get, and store it under the skin and at the stomach. This is one culprit for that bloated look.

Not good when trying to achieve a trim waistline!

The simple way to combat water retention is, not to avoid drinking water, but to chug it like it's going out of fashion. Your body's a smart cookie. (Someone say cookie...?) If your body knows it's getting all the water it needs, it has no reason to hang onto any, and make you suffer by looking like you swallowed a rubber ring.

How Much?

For decades, leading fat loss specialist Ellington Darden, PhD has been experimenting with the effects of water consumption on weight loss, which he's now culminated into a system he calls, "Super Hydration".

Super Hydration is a process of keeping the body well hydrated by drinking large quantities of ice-cold water. We've already discussed the benefits of drinking lots of water, but why ice cold?

Imagine, if you will, a food which actually has a caloric value equivalent to a minus number. You eat it, you *burn* calories...

Ice-cold water is that Holy Grail!

When you drink water that's ice cold, your body uses a certain amount of calories heating that water to core body temperature. For your body to heat one 300ml glass of ice-cold water, it will burn around 16 calories. Not much really. But if you drink 10, that's 160 calories. Do this every day, and by the end of the week, you'll have burned over 1,100 calories!

That's just by drinking water.

Now, you're probably thinking that 10 lots of 300ml – 3 litres - is a lot of water. And you'd be right. But it's not as out of reach as it seems.

Following the Super Simple Eating principle of eating little and often, let's say we're eating five times per day – three main meals and two snacks. Have one 300ml glass of water with every meal, and one in between each meal and you're there like swimwear.

That's it. That's all it takes!

And just by doing that, you've now added another layer to your "Success Stack".

Another great trick you can use, courtesy of Dr D, is to get a 500ml water bottle then stick six elastic bands around the body. Sip from the bottle throughout the day, and every time you drink a full bottle, all you do is move the band up from the body to around the neck. That way you always know how much you've drunk, *and* you have a visual goal to reach.

And – because I know you're thinking it – yes, you'll probably pee a lot! At least early on. But like the incredibly adaptive machine your body is, your bladder will get used to it after a week or so, and instead of nature calling every five seconds, it'll call less often but you'll spend longer on the phone.

If you get my drift.

Chapter 11

Super Simple Meals

"I cook with wine. Sometimes I even add it to the food."

– W.C Fields

I'll tell you now, I'm no Gordon Ramsey. I personally have all the cooking prowess of an arthritic chimpanzee. Keeping things simple isn't just a benefit to me, it's a necessity.

I've put together a handful of meals, made from a few ingredients thrown together and cooked in the most simple way. If you know how to sauté, flambé, or purée, then you fill your boots! But if you get by with a frying pan, a grill pan, and a microwave like me, you can still make great tasting, even fancy-pants looking meals quickly and simply.

Use these as a starting point when you're planning your meals. If you need more protein, for example, feel free to double up your serving size in your favourite meal. And don't forget, nutritionally, you can substitute any food with anything else from the same food group listed back in chapter 9.

Breakfast

Choc-nut Porridge

Microwave 40-50g (uncooked) of porridge oats (1 carb) with water.

Stir in a teaspoon of peanut butter (1 fat) and a scoop of chocolate whey protein (1 protein).

Scrambled Eggs

Slice a wholemeal English muffin (1 carb) and toast.

Top with a whole egg (1 fat) and 3-4 egg whites (1 protein), scrambled and seasoned with salt and pepper.

Salmon and Avocado Toast

Slice a wholemeal English muffin or sandwich thin (1 carb) and toast.

Spread thinly with low fat soft cheese, and top each half with ¼ of a mashed avocado (1 fat) and 80-100g of sliced salmon (1 protein).

Season to taste with salt and pepper and any other herbs your fancy.

Ham and Egg

Toast a crumpet (1 carb), and while toasting, poach an egg (1 fat).

Top crumpet with 2 slices of ham (½ protein) followed by the egg.

Nectarine and Berry Smoothie

Blend 1 nectarine (with stone removed), ¼ cup of frozen berries, and ½ a frozen banana (2 fruit), with 160ml of unsweetened almond milk or water, a teaspoon of ground cinnamon and a scoop of vanilla whey protein powder (1 protein).

Grape, Blueberry, and Chia Smoothie

Blend ½ cup of seedless grapes (red or green), ½ cup of frozen blueberries (2 fruit), 160ml of unsweetened almond milk or water, a teaspoon of chia seeds and a scoop vanilla whey protein powder (1 protein).

Lunch

Salmon Salad

Combine 2 handfuls of salad (the stuff pre-done in a bag works great for this - 1 veg) with a small dash of balsamic vinegar and a small dash of olive oil.

Top with 80-100g of sliced salmon (1 protein), and season to taste with salt and pepper.

Tortilla Pizza

Spread a mini tortilla wrap (1 carb) with tomato puree, add 80-100g of chopped pre-cooked chicken (or other lean meat or tuna – 1 protein), ½ cup of sliced mushrooms and ½ cup of finely chopped red onion (1 veg).

Top with a teaspoon of finely grated cheddar (1 fat).

Easy Ratatouille

Lightly fry a chopped onion and a chopped courgette.

Add a tin of chopped tomatoes (2 veg), a crushed clove of garlic and a dash of tomato purée.

Cover and simmer for around 20 minutes.

Season to taste and serve with 80-100g of a protein of your choice (works well with chicken, fish, tuna - 1 protein).

Mozzarella and Ham Salad

Place a handful of rocket, basil (to taste), and 4 halved cherry tomatoes (2 veg) in a bowl.

Top with ¼ of a chopped or sliced avocado (1 fat), 1 slice of torn mozzarella (1 fat) and 4 slices of ham (1 protein), and a drizzle of balsamic vinegar.

Mackerel and Lentils

Break 80-100g of cooked smoked mackerel (1 protein) into bite size chunks and heat.

Serve with ¼ of a sliced avocado (1 fat), a handful of halved cherry tomatoes and a cup of lamb's lettuce (3 veg), 50g of ready-cooked puy lentils (1 carb), and a handful of snipped fresh chives.

Drizzle with lemon juice, and a pinch of salt and pepper to taste.

Dinner

Chicken Satay

Heat 2 teaspoons of peanut butter (2 fat) in a saucepan with some water, a splash of soy sauce, a teaspoon of tomato puree, and a teaspoon of paprika.

Stir in 80-100g of pre-cooked chicken (1 protein) and heat through.

Serve with 80-100g of microwave pilau rice (1 carb), and 1-2 cups of mixed veg (1-2 veg).

Creamy Ham Spaghetti

Cook a serving of quick cook spaghetti (around 30g dry, or 80-100g fresh – 1 carb), and drain.

Stir in a dessert spoon of low fat soft cheese and 80-100g of chopped, cooked ham (1 protein).

Pasta Bolognaise

In a frying pan, brown off 80-100g of extra-lean beef mince or Quorn mince (1 protein) with a teaspoon of oil (1 fat).

Add a tin of chopped tomatoes and a sprinkling of Italian mixed herbs.

Simmer until the tomato juice has reduced and thickened, then serve with 80-100g of fresh spaghetti or pasta.

Paprika, Chicken, and Sweet Potato (serves 4)

Place 4 pieces of raw chicken (1 protein per serving), a red onion cut into wedges with a red and green pepper cut into chunks (1 veg per serving), and 300-400g of sweet potato chunks (1 carb per serving) in an oven-proof dish.

Sprinkle with paprika, and drizzle with 4 teaspoons of olive oil (1 fat per serving).

Bake for an hour and serve with a cup of salad per serving (1 veg per serving).

Dill and Tarragon Chicken

Heat 80-100g of pre-cooked chicken breast (1 protein) in a frying pan with a teaspoon oil (1 fat).

Add some chopped fresh or dried dill and tarragon and a tablespoon of low fat crème fraiche (1 fat).

Stir until all warm through and well combined, then serve with 80-100g of microwave rice (1 carb).

Cauliflower Cheese

Cook a small cauliflower (chopped) in a pan with water (2 veg), then split in two.

To one half, add 80-100g of cooked chicken (1 protein), a chopped, cooked bacon medallion (½ protein), and a cup of spinach, and place in an oven-proof dish.

Hand blend the other half of the cauliflower, add a teaspoon of grated parmesan cheese (1 fat) and stir.

Spoon on top of other ingredients. Cook for 30 mins in oven at 200 degrees.

Easy, Peasy Prawns

Heat 80-100g fresh spaghetti (1 carb), 1 cup of frozen peas (1 veg), and 80-100g of cooked frozen prawns (1 protein) in a pan of boiling water for around 3 minutes, and serve.

Inspiration
Melody Clarke

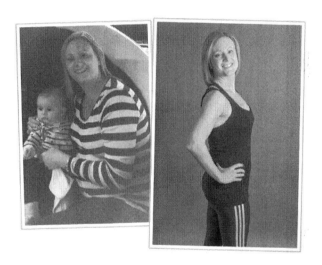

We've all heard it as mothers to be or new mums, it takes nine months to put the weight on and nine months to get the weight off. The trouble was that in January 2015, my daughter was nearing 7 months old and I was weighing 5lbs heavier than the week we'd returned from hospital.

Throughout my pregnancy I had been quite good, I'd tried hard not to eat for two as the thought of having to lose the baby weight was bad enough without adding to it by over eating. I'd never been any good at diets, I usually gave up after two weeks maximum, and never had the discipline to turn up to the gym or an exercise class two or three times a week. Plus I cancelled my gym membership when I found out I was expecting, and to be honest I was glad of the excuse not to go!

Throughout my teens and early 20's I was a slim thing and I quite enjoyed working out but as I got older, got my own house (and the responsibilities that come with it) and had a job with over an hour's commute each way, the gym was more of a chore than a pleasure and bad habits crept in. I'd talk myself out of going to the gym on the drive home or I'd get back too late to make any of the classes I liked, and so the weight piled on. I knew it was happening and I hated it but I wasn't disciplined enough to do anything about it. My life was too busy to fit in exercise. Slowly I had gone from a trim UK size 8 to an unflattering size 12-14 by the summer of 2012.

I was due to get married the following April on a beach in Mexico. I managed to lose 11lbs for my wedding but it took me 6 months and I was nowhere near as toned as I would have liked. I've always loved the sun and having a suntan, and I was going to wear a bikini no matter what, so I spent a lot of the holiday breathing in when all our friends and family were around!

It wasn't ideal and looking back I was disappointed in myself for not trying harder for my big day.

My daughter was born in June the following year and since her birth I had been eating what I liked when I liked telling myself that it was OK to eat cakes and biscuits to get by, or have a quick unhealthy lunch or evening meal as I was usually eating on the go, and to drink a glass of wine, or three, at the end of a tough day with the little one as a reward for getting through it. I wasn't happy having to choose loose fitting clothes or breathe in all the time. I wasn't happy looking at photos of myself with a double chin or looking almost twice the size of my friends but most of all I wasn't happy with the example I was setting my daughter.

In December a friend from my antenatal classes asked if I wanted to do a 28 day challenge with her in January, where she worked out at Anthony's transformation studio, so we could both start to shift our baby weight. At first I wasn't too keen as I knew it would be hard work and I didn't know if

I could stick to it for a whole 28 days. I'm a results driven person and if I don't see results or a change on the scales then I give up. Plus I had a house to run, a small baby to look after and very little spare time to fit in work out sessions. I knew my weight and appearance was depressing me but I justified it with the excuse that I'd just had a baby so it was ok to be carrying extra weight and have a wobbly tummy.

But she was getting older and that excuse was wearing thin!

When I stepped on the scales just after Christmas, the number displayed made up my mind that I needed to do the challenge and stop being in denial that I was happy with how I looked, baby or no baby.

I won't lie, it was tough! But as the days went on I got into my stride and learnt what were good and bad food choices by following the meal plans and guidance that was provided. As I started to see the numbers getting lower on the scales, it made me even more determined to do well. I learnt a lot about my attitude towards food and that I was actually quite lazy when it came to meal planning and cooking, relying on pasta dishes or ready meals as I didn't have the time or energy to cook when actually it doesn't take much to poach some chicken or fish and steam a few vegetables.

I don't have a support network around me who can look after my daughter whilst I work out, which was another excuse I had been dining out on for the previous 7 months, so it was invaluable to me and a huge part of my success that she was able to come with me to my workouts.

By the end of the 28 days I had lost 11lbs, the same amount it had taken me almost 6 months to lose for my wedding!

We went on our first family holiday in March and this time I wore my bikini feeling proud of the fact that I had a 9 month old baby and had done something about getting the baby weight off and getting myself back into good enough shape to start to feel confident about my body. But it didn't stop there, and I completed another 6 week challenge where I lost a further 12lbs, taking me back to the weight I was on my wedding day, except this time a lot more toned!

The new food and exercise regime in our house has also had a great effect on my husband who, in support of my latest challenge, completely changed his eating habits to eat what I was eating and he has seen a pretty substantial weight loss too! Now I feel like we're both setting our daughter a really good example and she has developed a much wider pallet by often eating the food off our plates!

I don't always make the workout sessions I plan to and it's not always easy to get out the house in the morning to get there but it's worth the effort to have my body and my confidence back. But even more than that, I feel proud of what I've achieved.

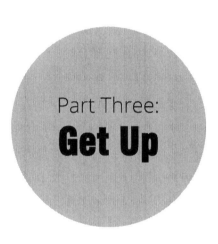

Part Three:
Get Up

Chapter 12

Intensity
vs
Time

"You have to stay in shape. My grandmother, she started walking five miles a day when she was 60. She's 97 today and we don't know where the hell she is."

– Ellen DeGeneres

Here's the million-pound question: exactly how long do we actually need to work out for to get results?

When my son was born, it wasn't fast, and it wasn't easy.

We had fantastic plans for a home-birth, got the pool, strung fairy lights up around the living room, and visualised a quick and easy labour followed by the appearance of a contented baby while a choir of angels sung lullabies over by the TV.

As it turned out, my son, Max had other ideas.

We should have been tipped off by the fact labour didn't even start until three weeks past his due date. He was pretty comfy in there, probably watching Friends re-runs with whiskey in one hand and a cigar in the other.

So instead of angels singing him into the world in our living room, labour took nearly three days and we were transferred to hospital. I suspect that was just as much because we'd exhausted the rota of midwives in the area as it was his stubbornness.

To cut a really, reeeeally long story short, in the end he had to be evicted via caesarean. Not quite what we'd planned, especially as I'd bribed the angel choir to sing "The Circle of Life" while I held him arms stretched to the window so all the commuters outside could bow in reverence.

Or something like that...

Anyway, the reason for the caesarean was that after the move to the hospital, my fiancée, Nic, and Max had both picked up an infection, so they basically had to get him out asap.

What that meant was that after the birth, they both had to stay in hospital for the next week while they were pumped full of antibiotics.

By this point you're probably wondering what this has to do with your workouts!

Well, from that first contraction through to being let out of the hospital was almost ten days. That's a long time for someone to be bent over birth pools and sleeping in hospital chairs!

That's me, by the way, not Nic...

My back didn't come out of that in the best shape, and a few weeks later, one of the discs in my spine finally gave up.

For several months I was walking on a crutch and taking enough medication to take down a small rhino, and in that time I blew up like the Michelin Man and became more and more unhappy by the day.

Despite being barely mobile, I had a business to run, so I was still working endless hours, then coming home at night wondering who'd stolen the hours from that day!

I was a mess.

Fat, twisted up like a pretzel, in a mild drug-induced haze most of the time, and exhausted.

I had spinal injections and threw myself into physio, and that's when I was smacked round the face with a huge dose of irony...

I was so busy, I couldn't even find time to attend one of my own 45 minute Bootcamp workouts!

I'd go days before I realised I hadn't worked out because between running my studio and spending all-important time with my family, time had just completely got away from me.

I knew what kind of results I *could* get. I see them every day in my members, and they're what inspire me to always raise my game. But once we've found time for work, for our kids, and our home lives... Once we've found time for *ourselves*, finding just an hour to cram in a workout is not just difficult, but often impossible!

And that was when I had my "Eureka!" moment. *TIME* is the problem!

So I did something a bit radical. I cut my Bootcamp workouts down from 45 minutes to 30 minutes, and guess what happened?

We started seeing even *better* results!

We even did an informal 'fitbit' test and had all our members in a couple of sessions track the calories burned, and it turned out we were burning over 30% more calories in the shorter sessions than we were in the 45 minute ones.

Like I said before, burning calories during the session isn't the goal. In fact it's a really poor reason for working out. But what it is is a good indication of how hard you're working - or in this case being worked.

So, like I said: How long do we actually *need* to work out to get results?

This is a question that's been asked over and over again since before exercise science was an actual science! And there is no definitive answer. But there have been several studies and what we do know is that if intense enough, as little as 4 minutes exercise can create an adaptation response.

Will that get you the best possible results? Not necessarily, but think about this - If you did nothing but a 4-minute workout that you knew would take you a little step further forwards six days out of every seven *consistently*, in three, six, twelve months from now you've just taken a LOT of steps forward!

On the other end of the scale, as we discussed right back in '*Set Up*', you can reach a point of diminishing returns if you work out for too long, and we also know now that the best results tend to happen in the first 30 minutes of a workout.

This is good news for you! Because, let's face it, when you're busy every second counts, and knowing you only need workout between 4 and 30 minutes to get results – that you don't need to lock yourself in the gym for even an hour, let alone several – is incredibly liberating.

But the key to these results is intensity. Effort.

In the simplest possible terms, the more effort you put in, the bigger the stimulus. The reason 4-minute workouts were shown to deliver were because of the effort put in.

Ever heard of Tabatas? They're an all-out effort for 20 seconds, alternated with rest periods of 10.

And the key words there are *all-out!* So we can keep the overall workout time down, but we need to work for it. And here's the clever bit...

There's a direct link between intensity and time. The harder you work, the less time you can sustain it for. You can't sprint a marathon, right?

So if you're really putting the effort in, not only *should* your workouts be shorter, but they *have to* be shorter.

So although a 4-minute workout may not be the absolute ideal to get the absolute best results, it's *enough* to create a stimulus that can move you forward. More importantly though, it's also enough to remove the barrier of *not* being able to work out, even on your busiest day, and remove the guilt that comes with missing a workout.

In reality, what you'll probably do is have a mix of workouts of different lengths depending on your situation on any given day - And for best results you *should*.

Chapter 13

HIIT vs MRT... What's with All the Acronyms?

"Everyone wants to win. But to truly succeed - whether it is at a sport or at your job or in life - you have to be willing to do the hard work..."

– Ronda Rousey

Everyone loves a good acronym, right? Nothing makes you feel more like a Secret Agent than reeling off some important sounding letters. CIA. FBI. Don't mess with me, I have a license to kill *and* a license to abbreviate.

Well, if you've ever picked up a workout magazine, you won't be left wanting!

HIT, HST, EDT, DTP... That's just a few workout styles that have their own initials, so you can feel like you're in a secret club while you're sweating it out.

Back in the early 00's, I was the Online Fitness Editor for Men's Health magazine. Every day that I logged on and trawled our reader message boards (we didn't have Facebook back then, and it was the best alternative to carrier pigeon) someone was asking about a "new" type of workout they wanted to try. And you can guarantee it had it's own acronym to describe it.

But the one just starting to come out of the woodwork was HIIT.

You've probably heard of HIIT. It's a bit of a buzz-word right now, and if you're not doing HIIT, you're just not one of the cool kids.

Innit.

The problem with HIIT is, it's also a bit of a catch-all term. An umbrella term if you like. There are a million and one ways you can do a HIIT workout, but not all of them will be the best way to strip the fat and sculpt and shape some lean, sexy muscle at the same time.

To do that we need to drill down a bit deeper. Give our workouts a much more laser-like focus.

So, I'm going to throw another cool sounding acronym at you:

MRT - Metabolic Resistance Training

See, there's one key element missing in a lot of HIIT workouts, and that's using movements which focus on building and toning lean, shapely muscle.

Want that tight waistline and lean looking abs? You need to focus on the muscle.

Want hot hips, and fabulous thighs? You need to focus on the muscle.

Want to swap out the bingo wings for toned triceps and upper arms? Guess what you need to focus on?

And that's where the resistance training comes in.

Resistance training is simply moving against a resistance. You don't even need weight for it, your own bodyweight can be that resistance. squats, pushups, dips, crunches... They're all resistance-type exercises.

So equipment should never be a barrier. A bit of floor space, and you're good to go.

You don't even need to have the latest workout gear, you can workout in your slippers if you like. I won't judge.

That being said though, we don't want to discount aerobic-type movements completely. We absolutely want to work some of those in too, but when you're throwing a workout together, around 80% of that workout should be resistance-type movements.

HIIT's OK, but too often than not can miss the mark. If you really want to be one of the cool kids MRT's where it's at.

Word.

Chapter 14

Workouts
That Work

"Wow, I really regret that workout!"

– Nobody. Ever.

Workouts, like your eating, should be super simple, and we're going to use just two simple protocols to get the job done.

Circuits

Don't think of these as circuits you do in a class at the gym, when you set up stations and move around them. This type of circuit you can do in one spot if you need to. No little picture cards necessary.

The key to having workouts that work *well* is doing the same or more work in *less* time. So if we're doing, say, 15 moves in 45 minutes, assuming we're performing those moves for the same period of time or the same number of repetitions, if we can do those same 15 moves in 30 minutes, that workout will get us better results. If we can do 20 moves in 30 minutes, that workout will probably be even more productive.

How do you cram more work into a shorter time period? Cut your rest times down. And a great way to do that is by stacking several exercises back-to-back.

So in a circuit you might do six exercises for 30 seconds each, and it might look like this:

1. Squat
2. Pushup
3. Ab Crunch
4. Mountain Climber
5. Inchworm
6. Plank

Set a timer to beep every 30 seconds (you can download an interval timer on your phone if you don't have one) then do them in sequence, no rest in between, changing at the beep.

Simple, right?

Circuits might have four exercises, they might have seven, but the important thing is they're performed with as little rest from start to finish as possible.

Don't get me wrong, if you haven't exercised for a while, or you're just starting out, you may need to stop a few times to catch your breath, or give your muscles a few seconds to stop screaming blue-murder. That's OK. But the goal remains the same:

Do as much as *you* can.

As you get stronger and fitter, you'll be able to keep going longer, and push yourself harder.

20/10s

Remember those Tabatas we talked about earlier? Well I like to do things a little differently. In the interests of doing more work in less time, that little 10 second rest period... Yeah, I've taken that out!

Instead, what I've found has worked really well is to alternate between two exercises, so you'll do 20 seconds of one exercise and 10 seconds of another. One thing we will keep intact though is, we'll still do eight total rounds which will last four minutes.

The real beauty in doing this is that we can apply these to a whole bucket-load of scenarios!

You want to spike your heart-rate? There's a 20/10 for that.

You want to give a particular body part a boost? Tighter tummy? Steely buns? There's a 20/10 for that.

You want to work loads of muscle in one short, concentrated, take-no-prisoners burst? There's a 20/10 for that.

It's the ultimate in flexibility and efficiency. In my studio we even dedicate an entire day of the week to 20/10s.

Here's a few examples of how you can stack these exercises to create workout epicness, first one being for 20 seconds, second one 10:

1. **Squat / Mountain Climber** - This combines a 'big' exercise like the squat with a cardio-focussed exercise for full-body conditioning in four minutes.

2. **Bicycle Crunch / Crunch-Hold** - We call this the "Gut Buster" in my training studio. This will fry your abs!

3. **Plank / Side Plank** - Simple but effective way to hit your core and pull in your waistline!

4. **Glute Bridge / One Legged Deadlift** - Laser target your bootay to strengthen, tighten, and tone!

Working alone or as part of a bigger workout, if you have a very small window to play with, then 20/10s are easily the best bang you can get for your buck.

Warm-Up

Some people have a "thing" they like to do that goes with their training. You know, some people like to do marathons. Some like to do triathlons. some just train to stay in shape and don't feel like they need to get up early on a Sunday to run around with a number pinned to their chest.

That's fine too.

My "thing" is Mudstacles. If you've never heard of this completely made-up word, it's the term used to describe obstacle courses that normally have you wading through mud and water at some point.

Something they've recently introduced to a lot of these is a group warm-up, where someone from one of the local gyms who've given them a wodge of cash to be put in front of the hundreds of people about to get up to their necks in mud, will stand on a little stage and get everyone doing star jumps at the start line.

The first time I experienced this was when I'd turned up for one of my favourite courses for, probably, the fourth time. We all got gathered ready to run, and before anyone knew what was happening, I found myself with everyone else unexpectedly doing Zumba in the middle of a field!

What has Zumba got to do with jumping fences and climbing cargo nets?

Nothing.

Literally nothing.

Now, don't get me wrong, before we get into the hard stuff, we *do* need to get your muscles moving and blood flowing, but warm-ups don't need to be elaborate, complicated, or... You know... Zumba!

We just need to raise your heart-rate a little bit, and get all the joints moving through a full range of motion to get blood-flow to all the major muscle groups and connective tissues, like your tendons and so-on.

This is the warm-up I use for most workouts in my studio, and will get your body ready for most types of MRT workout:

One Circuit, 30 seconds each exercise:

1. Pushups on your knees
2. Squat with Cross Crawl
3. Alternate Reverse Lunge with Torso Twist
4. Pushup-Row on your knees
5. Cross-Body Mountain Climbers

Then rest for 30 seconds before getting into your first circuit or 20/10.

If after that you feel you need a bit more warming up, or there are some muscles you feel need some more attention, then feel free to start your workout slow and build up. but don't fall into the trap of spending ages on an endless warm-up which ultimately becomes energy sapping and counter-productive.

Also notice that there isn't any stretching in the warm-up. That's by design. Research has shown that stretching a cold muscle is more likely to cause injury than prevent it, so stretching (unless you have a specific condition where you've been advised to stretch by a physio or other practitioner) is best left for the cool-down.

If you're doing a shorter workout because that's all you have time for, then you may choose to just take it easy and build up as you go. If your workout is just a 20/10, for example, the first three or four rounds you wouldn't be pushing yourself, then the last four or five you would go at it like a hungry kid in a pie shop. Always be careful though and listen to your body.

Cool Down

At the tail end of your workout, our muscles are burning, our heart's beating faster than a marching band on Red Bull, and we need to bring our body back down to Earth smoothly. This is when you want to go through a series of stretches.

Here I like to work from the top down. Truth be told, it doesn't matter too much what order you stretch your muscles in, but sticking to a sequence will help you make sure you don't miss anything out.

This is the progression I use as my go-to:

One circuit, hold for 15 seconds each:

1. Triceps Stretch (15 seconds on each arm)
2. Upper Back and Rear Shoulder Stretch
3. Chest and Front Shoulder Stretch
4. Standing Quadriceps and Hip Flexor Stretch (15 seconds on each leg)
5. Standing Hamstring and Calf Stretch (15 seconds on each leg)

If you have any particularly tight muscles, or if you've really focussed on one or two muscle groups more than others, feel free to spend a bit more time on them, or use a more specialised stretch. Otherwise, just those five simple stretches will be all you need to relax punished muscles and let your heart rate naturally come down.

Workout Scheduling

30 minutes of exercise five days per week. That's the Government's recommendation, and you've probably heard it or seen it on a leaflet at your local GP's. But we already know that just four minutes of the right type of exercise can get you results, and actually there's a bunch of research that says it doesn't really matter how often you workout, what's more important is that you workout consistently.

What I mean by that is that the person who works out twice-per-week, every week will get better results than the person who aims to work out five-times-per-week, but only gets there once one week, not at all the next week, four times the following week, and so on.

But whatever you do, I recommend you plan it in advance, whether that's for the month or for the week, put all of your workouts in your calendar as an appointment. We don't like to miss appointments so we're much less likely to miss a workout if it's in our diary.

Workout scheduling doesn't have to be complicated, just follow these super-simple guidelines:

- Two MRT workouts per week is great, three or four is better, five or more and you'll start to reach a point of diminishing returns.

- If your workouts are averaging 20 minutes or less, always have at least one day off per week. Two is better. You can do active-rest on these days.

- Don't go more than four days without working out. Remember, a 4-minute workout is *considerably* better than no workout.

- Don't do two workouts that specialise the same body parts on consecutive days, e.g. Monday - Abs, Tuesday - Abs, etc. But you can put two workouts that specialise different body parts back-to-back, e.g. Monday - Abs, Tuesday - Glutes (bum).

- Make sure you have at least one full-body workout with no particular body-part focus per week.

So, if you wanted to focus on your abs and glutes, your week's schedule might look like this:

Monday:	Full Body - 20 minutes
Tuesday:	Abs Specialisation - 4 minutes
Wednesday:	Full Body - 20 minutes
Thursday:	Rest Day
Friday:	Glute and Abs Specialisation - 30 minutes
Saturday:	Full Body - 30 minutes
Sunday:	Rest Day

Of course you don't need to plan your workouts on a 7-day rota if your life doesn't work that way. As long as you follow the basic rules laid out above, every week may be different for you and that's OK.

Off Days

Especially early on, when enthusiasm is spilling over like Katie Price's sports bra it's easy to want to workout every day. But rest is important too. In fact all the good stuff happens when you're resting!

How long you need to rest between workouts depends on a lot of things - How long your workout was, how hard your workout was, or even what body part or parts you were focussing on. They all play a part.

Although having at least one day of complete rest every week to ten days is good, you can also do 'Active Rest' on your off days. Active Rest is basically low-energy work such as going for a walk, or doing some stretching or foam rolling. It might be going to yoga, or throwing a frisbee with your kids.

The best description I've heard for active rest is, "...where you feel *better* after exercising compared to *before* you started". So if it's something that tires you out or leaves you breathless, that's not active rest.

That's exercise.

Chapter 15

Burn, Baby, Burn

"Greatness is a lot of small things done well. Day after day, workout after workout, obedience after obedience, day after day."

– Ray Lewis

Playlist ready? Trainers laced? Great. It's time to get moving.

On the next several pages I'm going to arm you with enough workouts to fill... well... a book!

I'm going to do something a little different too.

I've not designed workouts specifically for this book. Instead I've gathered together the exact circuits and 20/10s I've used that have produced the best results. Workouts that have been tried, tested, and proven in the real world.

Think of these like puzzle pieces. Just slot them together to make complete workouts to fit your situation.

For shorter workouts, you can do just one or two circuits or 20/10s, resting for 30 seconds in between.

For longer workouts (20-30 mins), here's some never-miss workout templates to plug the circuits and 20/10s into. By plugging the circuits and 20/10s listed later on into these templates, you have an almost unlimited amount of combinations to make workouts from:

1.
- Circuit 1
- 30 secs rest
- Circuit 2 or repeat Circuit 1
- 60 secs rest
- 20/10

2.
- Circuit 1
- 30 secs rest
- 20/10
- 30 secs rest
- Circuit 2

3.
- 20/10
- 30 secs rest
- 20/10
- 30 secs rest
- Circuit 1

4.
- Circuit 1
- 30 secs rest
- Circuit 2 or repeat Circuit 1
- 60 secs rest
- 20/10
- 60 secs rest
- 20/10

5.
- 20/10
- 60 secs rest
- Circuit 1
- 30 secs rest
- Circuit 2 or repeat Circuit 1
- 60 secs rest
- 20/10

6.
- Circuit 1
- 30 secs rest
- Repeat Circuit 1
- 60 secs rest
- 20/10
- 60 secs rest
- Circuit 2
- 30 secs rest
- Repeat Circuit 2

7.
- Circuit 1
- 30 secs rest
- Repeat Circuit 1
- 60 secs rest
- 20/10
- 60 secs rest
- Circuit 2
- 30 secs rest
- Repeat Circuit 2

8.
- 20/10
- 60 secs rest
- Circuit 1
- 30 secs rest
- Repeat Circuit 1
- 60 secs rest
- Circuit 2
- 30 secs rest
- Repeat Circuit 2

9.
- Circuit 1
- 30 secs rest
- Repeat Circuit 1
- 60 secs rest
- Circuit 2
- 30 secs rest
- Repeat Circuit 2
- 60 secs rest
- 20/10

10.
- 20/10
- 60 secs rest
- 20/10
- 60 secs rest
- 20/10
- 60 secs rest
- 20/10

11.
- 20/10
- 60 secs rest
- Circuit 1
- 30 secs rest
- Circuit 2
- 30 secs rest
- Circuit 3
- 60 secs rest
- 20/10

12.
- 20/10
- 60 secs rest
- 20/10
- 60 secs rest
- Circuit 1
- 30 secs rest
- Circuit 2 or repeat Circuit 1

13.
- Circuit 1
- 30 secs rest
- Repeat Circuit 1
- 60 secs rest
- 20/10
- 60 secs rest
- 20/10
- 60 secs rest
- Circuit 2
- 30 secs rest
- Repeat Circuit 2

14.
- Circuit 1
- 30 secs rest
- Repeat Circuit 1
- 60 secs rest
- Circuit 2
- 30 secs rest
- Repeat Circuit 2
- 60 secs rest
- Circuit 3
- 30 secs rest
- Repeat Circuit 3

Note: These are just the meat of the workout. Don't forget to warm up and cool down as described earlier on in Get Up.

Super Circuits

These circuits have either 6 or 7 exercises in them, and should be done for 30 seconds each. This makes each circuit 3-3½ minutes, which is just long enough to push yourself without having to start pacing yourself.

I've titled them with the main objective of each circuit.

1. **Full-Body**
   - 3-Stop Wide Squat (feet about 6 inches wider than usual)
   - Wide Squat Hold
   - Mountain Climber
   - 3-Stop Wide Pushup (hands about 3-4 inches wider than normal)
   - Plank
   - Cross-Body Mountain Climber
   - Inchworm

2. **Full-Body**
   - Prisoner Squat Crosscrawl
   - Mountain Climber
   - Side Plank with Hip Dip
   - T-Pushup
   - Side Plank with Hip Dip (other side)
   - Alternating Pushup-Superman
   - Spiderman Climb

3. **Strength**

- One-Legged Deadlift
- Woodchop
- Offset-Pushup (15 secs then change side)
- One-Legged Deadlift (other leg)
- Woodchop (other side)
- Pushup-Row
- Pushup-Hold

4. **Strength and Conditioning**

- Knee to Elbow Reverse Lunge (one side)
- Mountain Climber
- Knee to Elbow Reverse Lunge (other side)
- Spiderman Plank
- Prisoner Squat Crosscrawl
- Spiderman Climb
- Glute-Bridge Hold

5. **Conditioning and Core**

- Prisoner Squat
- Mountain Climber
- Traversing Pushup
- Plank with Hip Dip
- Prisoner Squat Crosscrawl
- Spiderman Climb
- Spiderman Plank

6. **Complete Core**

- Inchworm-Pushup
- Knee Cross
- Knee Cross (other side)
- Bicycle Crunch (one side only)
- Bicycle Crunch (other side only)
- Negative Clam Crunch

7. **Upper Body and Core**

- Side Plank with Crunch
- T-Pushup
- Side Plank with Crunch (other side)
- Bridge Crunch
- Glute Bridge Hold (both feet down)
- Ab Crunch Hold

8. **Upper Body and Core**

- Knee cross
- Pushup Row (row on one side)
- Knee cross (other side)
- Pushup Row (row on other side)
- Pushup to plank
- Clam crunch

9. **Upper Body**

- Side Plank with Crunch/Hip-Dip Combo
- Pushup-Superman
- Side Plank with Crunch/Hip-Dip Combo (other side)
- Plank with Alternate Leg Lift
- Grasshopper Plank
- T-Pushup
- Inchworm

10. **Upper Body**

- Squat (Feet about 6 inches wider than usual)
- Spiderman Plank
- Squat
- Grasshopper Plank
- Ski Squat
- Plank
- Bicycle Crunch (short and fast)

11. **Conditioning and Abs**

- Inchworm-Pushup
- Grasshopper Plank
- Cross-Body Mountain Climber
- Bicycle Crunch
- Ab Crunch
- Ab Crunch Hold

12. **Abs and Core**

- Bridge Crunch
- Side Plank with Crunch
- Alternate Superman
- Side Plank with Crunch (other side)
- Flutter Kick
- Bicycle Crunch

13. **Abs and Core**

- 3-Stop Ab Crunch
- Spiderman Plank
- Pushup-Superman
- Clam Crunch
- Grasshopper Plank
- Inchworm

14. **Abs**

- Bicycle Crunch (one side only)
- Ab Crunch
- Bicycle Crunch (other side only)
- TT-Crunch
- Reverse Crunch
- Bridge Crunch

15. **Abs**

- Oblique Crunch
- Knee Cross
- Inchworm Pushup
- Oblique Crunch (other side)
- Knee Cross
- Inchworm-Superman
- Grasshopper Plank

16. **Lower Body**

- Reverse Lunge
- Split Squat (same leg)
- 3-Stop Squat
- Reverse Lunge (other leg)
- Split Squat (other leg)
- Negative Squat
- Mountain Climber

17. **Lower Body**

- Prisoner Reverse Lunge
- Prisoner Split Squat (one leg)
- Travelling Mountain Climber
- Prisoner Reverse Lunge (other leg)
- Prisoner Split Squat (other leg)
- Travelling Mountain Climber
- Low Squat Hold

18. **Glutes and Core**

- Prisoner Squat
- Pushup-Superman
- Prisoner Alternate Reverse Lunge
- Glute Bridge
- Side Plank with Toe Tap
- Glute Bridge (other side)
- Side Plank with Toe Tap (other side)

19. **Glutes and Thighs**

- Wide Squat (Feet about 6 inches wider than usual)
- Glute Bridge
- Knee to Elbow Reverse Lunge
- Glute Bridge (other side)
- Knee to Elbow Reverse Lunge (other side)
- Ski Squat
- Mountain Climber (fast)

20. **Glutes**

- One-Legged Deadlift
- Kickout (same leg)
- Glute Bridge Hold (same leg)
- One-Legged Deadlift (other side)
- Kickout (other side)
- Glute Bridge Hold (other side)
- Negative Glute Bridge (both feet down)

Targeted 20/10s

Like poached eggs on warm, buttery toast, the magic of 20/10s is all in the exercise pairings. You can nail almost any objective with just two exercises. Here's 20 of my favourites to get you started.

1. **Full Body Conditioning**

   - Negative Pushup
   - Negative Squat

2. **Full body**

   - Touchdown Reverse Lunge
   - Pushup

3. **Conditioning**

   - Split Squat
   - Squat Thrust

4. **Upper Conditioning**

   - Pushup Row
   - Squat Thrust

5. **Upper Body and Core**

   - T-Pushup
   - Side Plank with Crunch

6. **Upper Body Taper**

   - Inchworm
   - Plank

7. **Sexy Shoulders**

   - Inchworm-Pushup
   - Pushup to Plank

8. **Arm Sculpting**

   - Close-Grip Pushup
   - Plank

9. **Arm and Ab Sculpting**

   - Superman Crunch
   - Negative Pushup

10. **Ab Sculpting**

    - Bicycle Crunch
    - Hold in Crunch Position

11. **Ab Sculpting**

    - Clam Crunch
    - Negative Crunch

12. **Tight Waistline**

    - Side Plank with Hip Dip
    - Knee Cross

13. **Tight Waistline**

    - Cross-Body Mountain Climbers
    - Side Plank

14. **Lower Conditioning**

    - Knee to Elbow Reverse Lunge
    - Squat Thrust

15. **Triceps and Glutes**

   - Spiderman Pushup
   - Close-Grip Pushup

16. **Glute and Core Sculpting**

   - Side Plank with Toe Tap
   - Plank with Alternate Leg Lift

17. **Glutes, Legs, and Core**

   - Prisoner Squat Crosscrawl
   - Traversing Pushup

18. **Glute Sculpting**

   - Glute Bridge
   - One-Legged Deadlift

19. **Lean Legs**

   - Squat
   - Hold in Low Squat Position

20. **Lean Legs**

   - 3-Stop Split Squat
   - Negative Squat

Chapter 16

Do-Anywhere
Fat-Busting Moves

"I like to move it, move it. I like to move it, move it. I like to move it, move it. Ya like to move it."

– Reel 2 Real

These are what I consider to be the best of the best body-shaping, fat-busting moves. You can workout with dumbbells, barbells, or fancy machines, and while they're all useful tools, the truth is you don't need any of them to sculpt your perfect body.

All you need is exactly that: Your body.

So these moves I've gathered together can be done pretty much anywhere, any time, in whatever you're wearing. Unless you're wearing a space-suit. But, hey, what you do on your own time...

Bad-arse as they are, before we get into the exercises, let's talk about performance.

Exercises don't always have to be up and down. When you squat, you don't have to just go: Squat down, stand up, squat down, stand up, etc. While most exercises will be done like this, there are other techniques we can use to squeeze extra awesomeness out of some movements. If you've already had a look through the example circuits and 20/10s, you'll have probably spotted a few of them subtly sprinkled in like a ninja in a room full of nuns.

Two of my favourite ways to crank up the intensity of an exercise is to use Isometrics and Negatives.

Isometrics

This is just a fancy word for holding an exercise in a certain position. In a lot of cases, you'd hold it in the fully contracted position. So in a squat it would be in the bottom position when your thighs are roughly parallel to the floor, or in a pushup, when your arms are at around or slightly below 90 degrees. But really you can experiment with where in the movement you're going to stop and smell the roses for a bit.

Isometrics are effective because you are at your strongest in a static position. I.e. you can hold in a static position more weight than you could lift through a full range of motion.

What that means is, if you can't (for example) do a full pushup on your toes, chances are you can hold a low pushup position on your toes.

So even when you're fatigued from doing normal pushups or other upper body exercises, you can probably squeeze out a little bit more effort by sticking in an isometric hold.

So if you see Squat Hold, Crunch Hold, Pushup Hold, Glute-Bridge Hold... Anything like that in one of the circuits or 20/10s, it just means rather than go up and down, you're going to hold the contracted position of that exercise for the allotted time. For example, in a squat or pushup hold the bottom position, in a glute bridge or crunch, hold the top position.

Negatives

The technical term for this is Eccentric. But despite the word 'negative' sounding like a bit of a downer, all it's really referring to is the lowering part of an exercise. So in a squat, it would be the squatting down part, not the standing up part (the positive).

During the lowering part of an exercise, we're around 40% stronger than the lifting part. So in practical terms, like isometrics, that means we can use negatives as a way to keep pushing when we're tired.

There's two ways you can approach negatives. One is just to really slow down in the negative part of a movement, so if you had 30 seconds of negative squats, you'd go really slow on the way down, then push back up and repeat for 30 seconds. So you might do three reps with a 10 second negative, or two reps with a 15 second negative. These are called Negative Accentuated reps.

The other way is to take your designated time and try to move so slowly you do one rep in that time. So if you have a 30 second set, you'll aim to take 30 seconds from top to bottom.

Negatives take a lot of control and can take practice, but by slowing down when you're stronger (lowering), you can really lower the amount of momentum you're using and create more tension in the target muscles.

3-Stop Reps

And on that note of taking out momentum, another great way to get this done is to work short isometric holds right into the negative movement.

In most movements, you can comfortably get in three full-stops before the movement just becomes a series of micro-movements, so 3-stop reps are the perfect way to get the best of both worlds.

Using our trusty squat again, starting at the top, you'd go down a little bit, then pause for a second or two. Go down a bit more, pause again.

Then go down one more time, pause at the bottom, than push up back to the start and repeat.

That way, you never really get the chance to build momentum on that downward movement, so your muscles have to work that bit harder.

Complex Movements

Think of these as combo-movements. Two movements stacked on top of each other.

This could be an Inchworm-Pushup – walking down on your hands into plank position, then before walking back up doing a pushup. It might be a Pushup-Superman – after pushing up, lifting and lowering one leg and the opposite arm before doing your next pushup.

These work really well as a way to get more bang for your buck by working more muscles in the same period of time.

All of these things not only add variety, but can add intensity to your workout. And the bottom line is, if you can work that little bit harder, your results will be that little bit better.

One Legged Deadlift

- Stand on one leg with your hands out in front of you for balance, and your other leg bent behind you.

- Bend the knee of your stationary leg pushing your bottom back and extending your free leg out behind you for balance.

- Continue lowering as far as you can comfortably, and then return to the upright position driving forward with your hips.

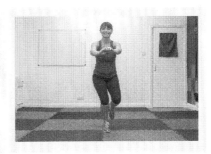

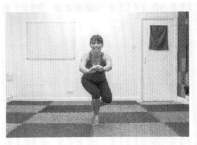

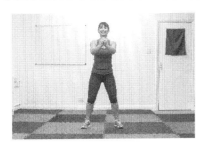

Squat

- Start by standing with your feet a little wider than shoulder width apart, your arms out in front of you, and your knees slightly bent.

- Squat down as far as you can comfortably by pushing your bum back, and keeping your weight through your heels.

- Keeping your core in tight and your chest up, stand back up to the starting position, and repeat.

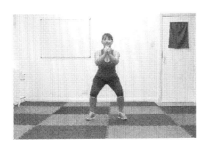

Ski Squat

- Stand with your feet about six inches apart and your hands out in front of you.

- Push your bum back, and squat down as far as you can comfortably, being careful not to let your knees collapse inwards as you get lower.

- Push through your heels to come back up to standing, and repeat.

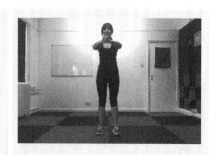

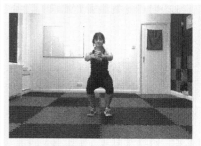

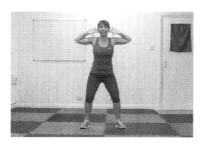

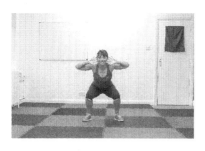

Prisoner Squat

- Start by standing with your feet a little wider than shoulder width apart, your knees slightly bent, and your hands beside your head.

- Keeping your shoulder blades squeezed together, squat down as far as you can comfortably by pushing your bum back, and keeping your weight through your heels.

- Keeping your core in tight and your chest up, stand back up to the starting position, and repeat.

Split Squat

- Start by standing with your feet about 6 inches apart, your hands on your hips, then take a big step backwards.

- Squat down, dropping the back knee as far as you can without touching the floor.

- Keeping your core in tight and your chest up, stand back up to the starting position, pushing through your front heel, and repeat.

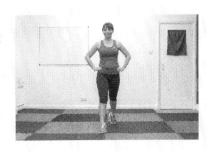

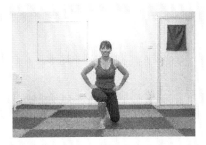

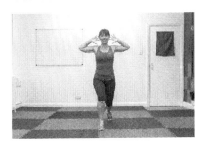

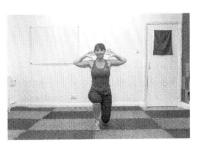

Prisoner Split Squat

- Start by standing with your feet about 6 inches apart, your hands beside your head, then take a big step backwards.

- Squat down, dropping the back knee as far as you can without touching the floor.

- Keeping your core in tight and your chest up, stand back up to the starting position, pushing through your front heel, and repeat.

Prisoner Squat Crosscrawl

- Stand with your feet a little wider than shoulder width, and your knees slightly bent.

- Place your hands behind your head and pull your elbows back to squeeze your shoulder blades a little.

- Bend your knees down into a squat, then as you come back to standing, lift one knee up to your chest, rotating your upper body towards that knee.

- Return to starting position and repeat, alternating legs.

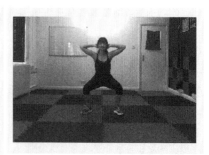

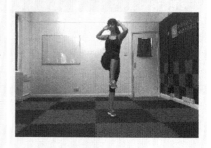

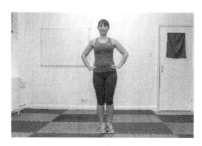

Reverse Lunge

- Start by standing with your feet about 6 inches apart and your hands on your hips.

- Take a large step backwards with your left foot.

- Lower your hips to the floor, bending your back knee towards the floor and keeping your front leg at a 90-degree angle.

- Push through the front heel to return to the starting position, and repeat either on the same leg, or alternating legs.

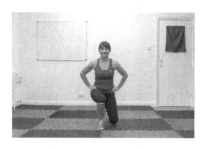

Prisoner Reverse Lunge

- Start by standing with your feet about 6 inches apart and your hands beside your head.

- Take a large step backwards with your right foot.

- Lower your hips to the floor until your front (left) knee forms a 90-degree angle.

- Push through the front heel to return to the starting position, and repeat either on the same leg, or alternating legs.

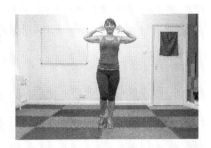

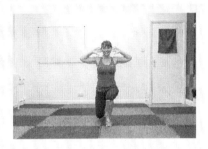

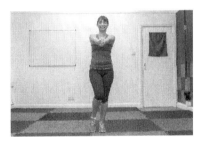

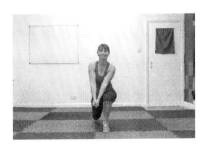

Touchdown Reverse Lunge

- Start by standing with your feet about 6 inches apart and your hands out in front clasped together.

- Take a large step backwards with your right foot.

- Bending your front leg 90-degrees, bring both arms down towards the inside ankle of your front leg in a chopping motion.

- Push through the front heel to return to the starting position, and repeat either on the same leg, or alternating legs.

Knee to Elbow Reverse Lunge

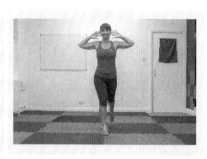

- Start by standing with your feet together, your knees slightly bent, and your hands beside your head.

- Keeping your shoulder blades squeezed together, step back on one leg.

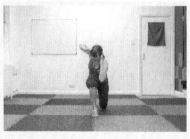

- Drop the back knee down, and at the same time, while keeping your core tight, rotate the opposite elbow down towards the front knee.

- Push through the front heel to return to the starting position, and repeat either on the same leg, or alternating legs.

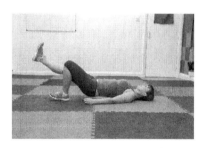

Glute Bridge

- Lie on your back with your hands by your side, one leg bent, and the other in the air.

- Start by tucking your tail bone under and pulling your core in so your lower back is flat against the floor, then, pushing your heel down and squeezing your glutes, lift your bum up and back as far as you can.

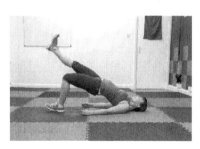

- Slowly lower to the floor, then repeat.

- This can also be done with both legs on the floor.

Kickout

- On the floor get down onto your hands and your knees.

- Lift your right leg and bring the knee in towards your left elbow.

- Push your right leg back into a 90-degree angle so your heel is pointing towards the ceiling.

- Return to the starting position and repeat with the same leg, or alternate legs.

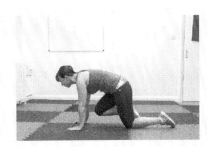

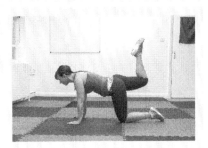

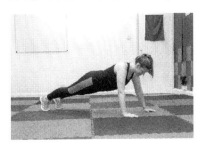

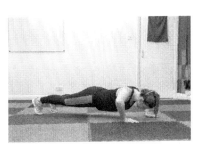

Pushup

- Face the floor with your hands down, arms extended and up on your toes.

- Position your shoulders over your wrists and your body in a straight line from head to toe.

- Bend your elbows and lower your chest towards the floor going down as far as you can.

- Push back up to the starting position.

- To simplify this exercise put both knees on the floor or lean against a wall.

Close-Grip Pushup

- Get into pushup position and place your hands under your chest closer than shoulder width apart.

- Keeping your elbows in tight to your body, lower yourself down to the floor bending your elbows as far as you can.

- Straighten your elbows and push yourself back up to the starting position.

- To simplify this exercise put both knees on the floor or lean against a wall.

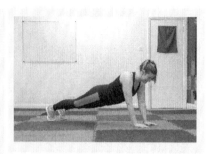

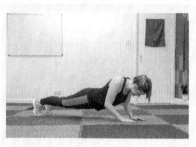

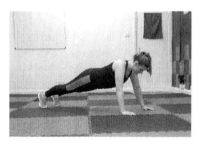

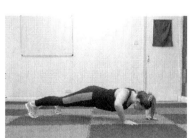

Grasshopper Pushup

- Start by getting into a pushup position, with your core tight and hands wide.

- Step one foot out to the side, keeping that leg straight, then lower your upper body down into a pushup.

- Push back up to the starting position, then repeat with the other leg.

- Do this with your knees down, straightening the leg out to the side if you need to make it easier.

Offset Pushup

- Start by getting into a pushup position with your hands slightly wider than normal, then move one hand a couple of inches forward, and the other a couple of inches back.

- Keeping your core in tight, slowly lower your chest to the floor, then push back up and repeat.

- Do this with your knees down if you need to make it easier.

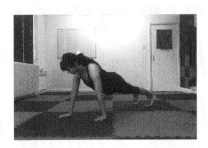

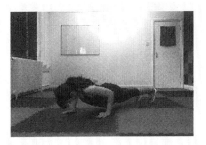

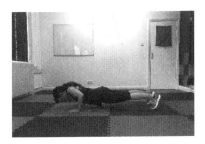

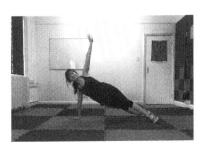

T-Pushup

- Start by getting into a pushup position, with your core tight and hands wide.

- Slowly lower down, then as you push back up, roll over to one side, reaching up to the ceiling.

- Carefully return to the pushup position and repeat.

- If you want to make this harder, when you rotate up, you can stack your feet into a full side plank position.

Pushup Row

- Get into pushup position.
- Bend your elbows and lower your chest towards the floor going down as far as you can.
- Push back up to the starting position.
- Once you're back in the starting position, clench your right fist and make an upwards pulling motion with your right arm pointing your elbow up towards the ceiling.
- Return to the staring position and repeat with the left arm.

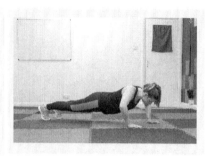

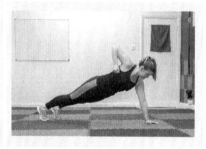

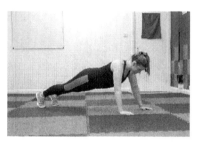

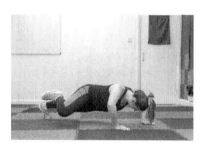

Spiderman Pushup

- Get into pushup position.
- Lift your right leg off the floor and bring your knee around the outside of your body towards your right elbow.
- As you bring your knee towards your elbow, bend both elbows and lower your chest towards the floor at the same time, going down as far as you can.
- Return to the starting position and repeat with the other leg.
- To simplify this exercise put both knees on the floor.

Traversing Pushup

- Get into pushup position.

- Bend your elbows and lower your chest towards the floor going down as far as you can.

- Push back up to the starting position.

- Traverse sideways by bringing your hands together, while stepping out to the side with the opposite leg.

- Repeat by pushing up again, then traversing back in the other direction.

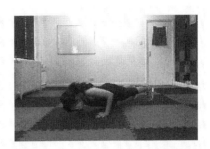

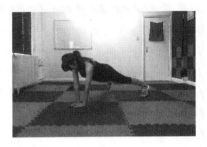

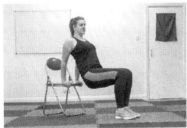

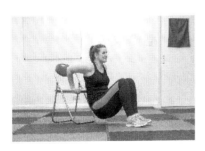

Tricep Dip

- Position your hands shoulder-width apart on a stable chair.

- Bend your legs to 90-degrees and keep your arms straight.

- Slowly bend your elbows to lower your body towards the floor until your elbows are at about a 90-degree angle.

- Push back up until your elbows are nearly straight. Do not lock them.

- Straighten your legs to make this harder.

Plank

- Get into pushup position.

- Bend your elbows and rest your weight ono your forearms.

- Your body should form a straight line from shoulders to ankles.

- Suck your belly button into your spine about 30% keeping your head up.

- Hold this position.

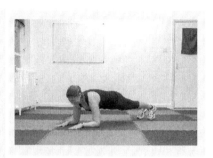

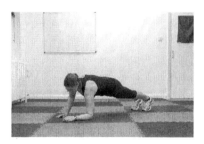

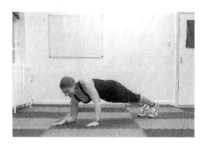

Pushup to Plank

- Get into pushup position.

- Bend your elbows one at a time to rest your weight ono your forearms.

- Keeping your core tight and your bottom down, push back up with your hands, extending your arms one at a time to get back into pushup position then repeat.

Plank with Hip Dip

- Start by getting into a plank position, either on your elbows or hands.

- Keeping your core in tight, rotate your hips to one side as far as you can, so one hip is aiming for the floor.

- Pull your core in and return to the start position.

- Repeat to the other side.

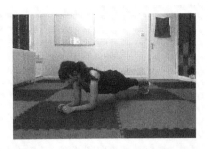

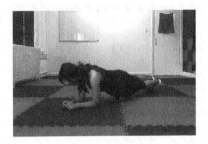

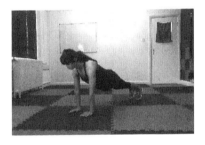

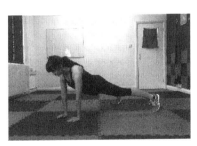

Grasshopper Plank

- Start by getting into a plank position, either on your elbows or hands.

- Keeping your core in tight, step one foot out to the side, keeping that leg straight.

- Tap it down to the floor, then return to the starting position.

- Repeat to the other side.

- Do this with your knees down, straightening the leg out to the side if you need to make it easier.

3-Point Plank

- Get into a plank position.

- Raise your left leg, bending at the knee into a 90-degree angle so the bottom of your foot is pointing towards the ceiling.

- Hold.

- Return to your starting position and repeat with the other leg.

- You can also pulse the leg that's up by making little pushes towards the ceiling for added glute focus.

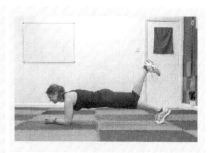

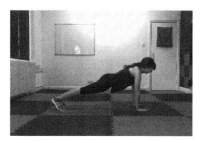

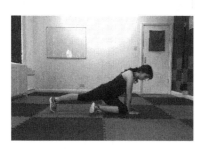

Knee Cross

- Start by getting into a plank position on your hands.

- Keeping your core in tight, rotate your hips, bringing your knee through and under your body towards the opposite hand.

- Return to the starting position, without touching your toes down, and repeat.

Spiderman Plank

- Get into pushup position.
- Your body should form a straight line from shoulders to ankles.
- Keeping your core tight, lift your right leg off the floor and bring your knee around the outside of your body towards your right elbow.
- Return to the starting position and repeat with the other leg.
- Drop to your elbows and/or knees to make this easier.

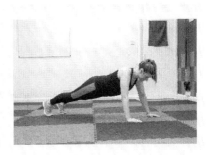

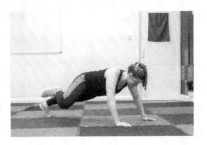

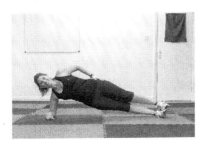

Side Plank

- Lie on your side with your feet together and one forearm at 90-degrees directly below your shoulder.
- Place your top foot on top of your bottom foot and hold the position.
- To simplify this exercise bend your bottom.
- To make it harder, pushup onto your hand and lift your upper arm straight above your head.

Side Plank with Leg Raise

- Lie on your side with your feet together and one forearm at 90-degrees directly below your shoulder.
- Place your top foot on top of your bottom foot.
- Lift your upper leg towards the ceiling creating a V shape with your legs and hold the position.
- To simplify this exercise bend your bottom knee.
- To make it harder, pushup onto your hand and lift your upper arm straight above your head.

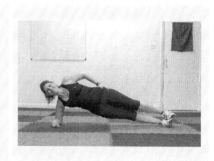

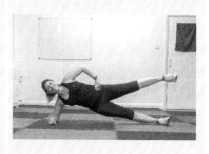

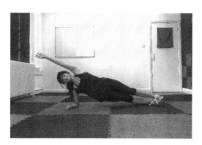

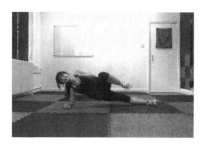

Side Plank with Crunch

- Start by getting into a side plank position either on your elbow or hand, then extend your top arm over your head.
- Keeping your core in tight, bend your arm down and your knee up to meet in the middle, squeezing your abs.
- Pause briefly and return to the starting position.
- Do this with your bottom knee down if you need to make it easier.

Side Plank with Hip Dip

- Lie on your side with your feet together and one forearm at 90-degrees directly below your shoulder, and your top foot on top of your bottom foot.

- Lower your hip towards the floor as far as you can without touching it, then lift back up.

- To simplify this exercise bend your bottom knee.

- To make it harder, pushup onto your hand and lift your upper arm straight above your head.

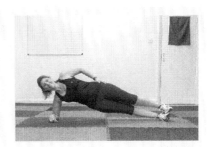

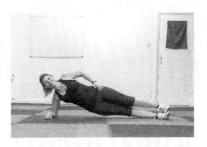

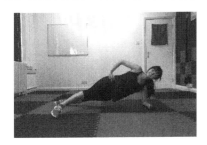

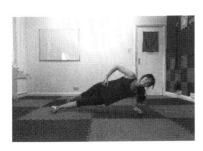

Side Plank with Toe Tap

- Start by getting into a side plank position either on your elbow or hand.

- Keeping the top leg straight, tap it down in front of your body.

- Bring the leg back to the centre line lifting it up high, then tap it down behind the body.

- Bring it back to the centre line again, and repeat.

- Bend your bottom knee if you need to make this easier.

Superman

- Get into pushup position.
- Lift your right arm and left leg so they are parallel with your body.
- Hold.
- To simplify this exercise go onto your knees.

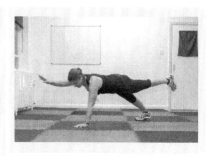

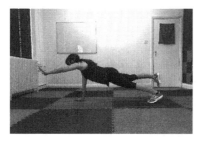

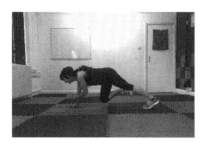

Superman Crunch

- Start in a plank position on your hands, then lift your left foot off the floor, and extend your right arm out in front of you.
- Keeping your core tight, bend your elbow and knee, bringing them together, then extend back to the start position and repeat.
- If you need to make this easier, you can do it on your hands and knees.
- This can be done on one side, or alternating.

Inchworm

- Place your hands on the ground in front of your toes in pushup position keeping your knees bent slightly.

- Walk your hands backwards pushing back with your bottom until your hands are close to your feet.

- Slowly walk your hands forwards and away from your body until your body is parallel to the ground back in a pushup position.

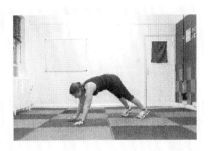

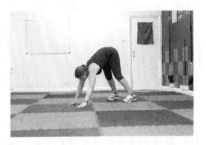

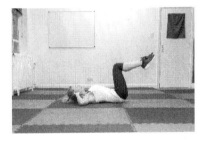

Ab Crunch

- Lie flat on the floor with your lower back pressed against the ground and your hands beside your head, then lift your knees to 90 degrees.

- Keeping a peach-sized gap between your chin and your chest, slowly curl your shoulders and shoulder blades off of the floor, trying to peel one vertebrae up at a time.

- Pause briefly at the top, then lower back to the ground.

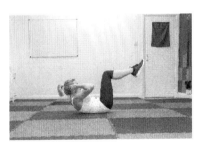

Bicycle Crunch

- Lie flat on the floor with your lower back pressed to the ground.
- Put your hands behind your head, bring both knees in towards your chest and lift your shoulder blades off the ground.
- Straighten your right leg out as far as you can while twisting your upper body to the right, bringing your right elbow towards the left knee.
- Alternately touch your elbows to the opposite knee twisting back and forth and keeping your elbows back and hands behind your head.

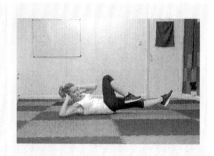

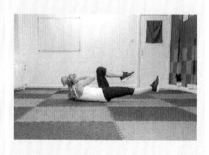

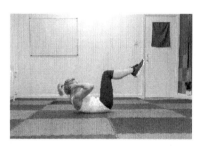

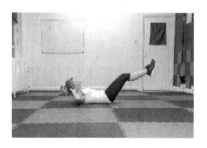

Clam Crunch

- Lie flat on the floor with your lower back pressed against the ground and your hands beside your head.
- Bring both knees in towards your chest and at the same time curl your upper body to meet your knees at a 90-degree angle.
- Reverse the movement, lowering your head and feet back down towards the ground as far as you can without your lower back lifting.

Bridge-Crunch

- Lie on your back with your feet hip width apart and your hands beside your head.

- Tuck your tail bone under, then lift your bum up towards the ceiling, while simultaneously pushing your heels down into the floor.

- Lower your bum back to the floor, then curl your shoulder blades off the floor into a crunch.

- Lower yourself back to the starting position, and repeat.

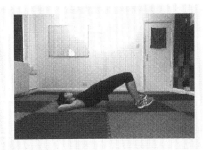

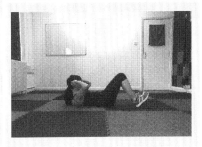

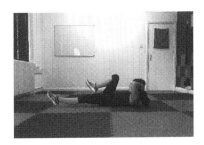

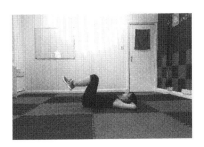

TT Crunch

- Start by lying on your back with your knees up at 90 degrees, your hands beside your head, and your shoulders curled off the floor.

- Keeping your lower back pushed against the floor, extend one leg and tap that heel down, come back to the start and repeat with the other leg, then come back to the start and lower your head and shoulders down to the floor for a crunch.

- Return to the starting position and repeat.

Oblique Crunch

- Lay on your back with your feet on the floor and your knees bent, then drop your knees down to one side and extend your arms out in front of you.

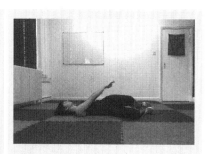

- Keeping your core pulled in, and your lower back pushed firmly against the floor, slowly peel your shoulders and shoulder blades off the floor, reaching your hands towards your heels.

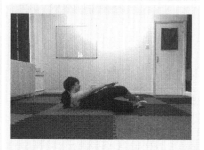

- Lower back to the start and repeat.

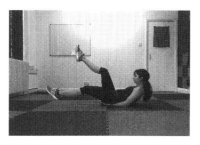

Flutter Kick

- Lie on your back and tuck your hands under the sides of your hips, pushing your lower back into the floor.

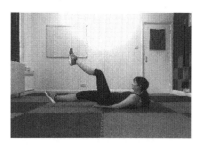

- Keeping a peach sized gap under your chin, lift your head and shoulders off of the floor, then keeping your knees slightly bent, lift your feet a few inches off of the floor.

- Lift one leg up towards the ceiling, then in a scissor motion, bring this leg back down while lifting the other leg, and repeat.

Woodchop

- Stand with your feet a little wider than shoulder width, your knees slightly bent, and your hands lightly clasped together.

- Rotating at the hips, bring your hands back and over your head to one side.

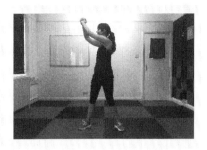

- Rotating at the hips again, bend your knees, bringing your hands down across the body to the other side knee in a smooth chopping motion.

- Return to the starting position, keeping your core tight throughout.

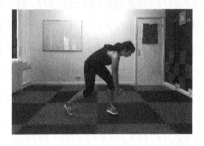

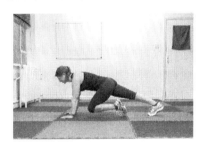

Mountain Climbers

- Get into pushup position.

- Keeping your core tight, pick up your right foot and bring your knee toward your right elbow.

- Bring your foot back to pushup position and repeat with your left foot towards your left elbow.

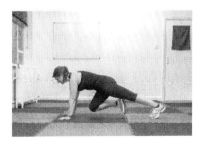

Cross-Body Mountain Climbers

- Get into pushup position.

- Keeping your core tight, pick up your right foot and bring your right knee toward your left elbow.

- Bring your foot back to pushup position and repeat with your left foot towards your right elbow.

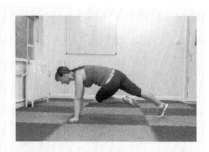

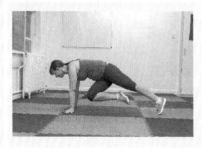

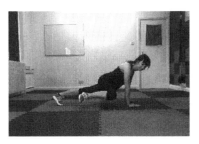

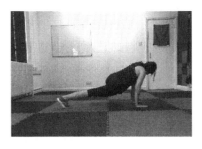

Travelling Mountain Climbers

- Start in a pushup position ready to do mountain climbers.

- Rotate your hips to one side, then do three mountain climbers.

- Rotate your hips back to centre, then do three more.

- Rotate your hips to the other side and do three more.

- Rotate your hips back to centre and repeat.

Spiderman Climb

- Get into pushup position.

- Lift your left leg off the floor and bring your knee around the outside of your body towards your right elbow, tapping your foot to the floor.

- Return to the starting position and repeat with the other leg.

- To simplify this exercise put both knees on the floor.

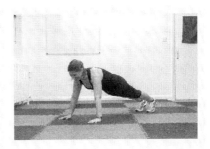

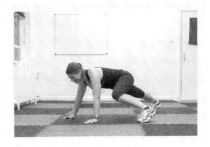

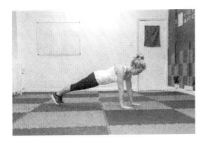

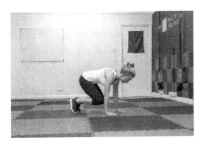

Squat Thrust

- Start in a pushup position with your hands about shoulder width apart, and your back straight.

- Bring your knees in towards your elbows with your hands remaining on the ground, staying light on your feet.

- Kick your feet back into pushup position keeping your hands on the ground.

Inspiration

Nicole Parker

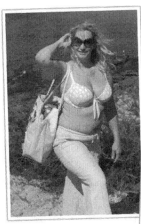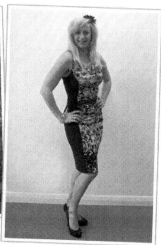

When I committed to get fit, I didn't mess about! I gave up smoking, and when my then boss asked if anyone wanted to join him for a marathon, I immediately said yes, even though I'd only ran a 5km race before then!

I did a half-marathon in preparation, and when I crossed the finish line and saw my training partner; I burst into tears on the spot saying, "How the hell am I going to do a full marathon?!"

But I did it! It was a really, really hot day, and I had to walk-run-walk-run a few miles in the middle, but I crossed the line in 6½ hours, and the experience was really amazing!

But all the time I was running, even though I was following advice regarding what I thought I should be eating, despite clocking up so many miles, I still didn't seem to be losing any weight at all.

The training had been so hard for the marathon and I had stayed in so much and been good with not drinking that after I finished the marathon, I fell off the wagon. I didn't go out running for about three months; I went out drinking quite a lot and ended up smoking a little bit more again. But then I stopped myself again because I knew I didn't want to lose the fitness that I'd gained.

My boyfriend at the time also mentioned to me I'd put on a bit of weight, which as a woman, and having it come from the person closest to you, was really hard to hear. However, ironically, he actually did me a big favour because it made me think, "Right, OK, I need to do something about this and make him fancy me again!" and if he hadn't done that, I probably wouldn't be where I am today.

I started a new job, and I'd seen the Anthony's Body-Transformation programme advertised and knew I'd be able to make it there in the morning now, before work. I signed up for that and started about a week after I had started my new job.

It's always very hard in the beginning to drag yourself out of bed, especially if you're not used to the early starts however, the moment you start seeing results, it just stops being a chore! And seeing the results just spurs me on to keep going.

I have quite a scientific brain and Anthony always explained to me a lot about the science behind resistance training. For example, if you have more muscle, you will naturally burn more calories, even at rest because muscles need more energy just to "be". He also dispelled the myth of "muscle weighs more than fat" and showed how compact muscles are, so of course you are going to be able to wear smaller sizes.

Although I was never really a very active person, I did always think that yes, having muscles would make a woman look more "manly" but again, Anthony proved to me time and time again that this was just not the case, especially using the science. It all just made so much SENSE to me - I still can't believe that this is not taught in schools or is not more common knowledge. To begin with, I was resistant but with Anthony's firm but encouraging coaching skills, I began to lift heavier and heavier and then I was getting smaller and smaller. And before I knew it, just day-to-day living was becoming easier - climbing stairs, lifting shopping etc. Why did I not know this secret before?!

I went into Debenhams the other day and bought three dresses in a UK size 10 and one in a size 8; I never thought, ever, that I'd be able to get into a size like that. I need to go shopping for a whole new wardrobe now because none of my old clothes fit me anymore!

I look at my "before" photos now and I never, ever want to get like that again. I don't think I ever will either because my whole mindset has changed – how I think about exercise and food and my relationship with it. For example, I've always eaten when I'm bored. I always need to be on the go and, when I stop, I used to start eating to fill the time; particularly at my old workplace. I was bored a lot of the time in that job and it was the kind of workplace where people brought in cakes all the time. I think in just the year I worked there I probably gained a stone of fat! It's no wonder my ex stopped fancying me!

My life change has been incredible. I walk down the street and I feel like a new woman. I feel amazing! It's really hard to put it into words because I feel like I'm just gushing about it all the time to other people! I just feel so happy; the happiest I've ever been and so super-duper confident. I've never really felt like this before and it's addictive!

What is also addictive is becoming an inspiration to other women. They ask me my "secret" and I tell them to start resistance training and interval training and to spread the word. Literally everyone needs to know about how it can be fun and not boring to train in this way and hey! Who doesn't want to feel and look like Wonder Woman?!

It's weird when you walk down the street and you notice people are staring! One time, three random men said good morning to me on my walk to work! I just have this new lease of life and if someone had told me at 22, "Nicole – in ten years' time you'll be a size 8-10 and you'd have already run two half marathons and a full marathon", I would have said, "Yeah, right!", and lit up another cigarette!

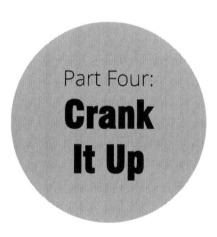

Part Four:
Crank It Up

Chapter 17

30 Ways to Stoke the Fire

"Greatness is a lot of small things done well. Day after day, workout after workout, obedience after obedience, day after day."

– Ray Lewis

Ever heard the saying pennies make pounds? Or the little things add up?

It's true you need to get the big things in order first – Eating right, doing the right type of exercise, etc. – but when you have those nailed down, the little additions can make a big difference.

So that in mind, here's 30 little things you can plug in to help you level up your results.

1. **Start the day with eggs:** Several studies of overweight women have shown that eating eggs for breakfast can increase weight loss by as much as 65% when compared to a carbohydrate based breakfast (as part of a calorie controlled diet).

2. **Start each meal with a glass of water:** Drinking water before meals can stop you mistaking hunger for thirst, and in one study helped people eat fewer calories and increase weight loss by 44%.

3. **Use water to kickstart your metabolism in the morning:** 1 glass of water, particularly as the first thing you have can increase metabolism by up to 30% for the next hour and a half.

4. **Use smaller plates:** We eat with our eyes (Masterchef focus on presentation for a reason!) and putting your food on smaller plates has been shown to fool us into thinking we're eating more and triggering our full response sooner.

5. **Keep a food diary:** In a study done on 1500 people, those who wrote down what they ate lost TWICE as much weight as those who didn't.

6. **If you're hungry, brush your teeth:** The tingling sensation has been shown to decrease hunger pangs, and the minty taste.

7. **Photograph your food:** Taking a photo of your food before eating it has been shown to increase weight loss even more than just writing down what you eat because it acts as an intervention at the time of eating, rather than retrospectively.

8. **Take a before photo:** And if you can strip down to your bathing suit. Then keep it where you can access it at any time. On your phone, in a draw in the kitchen. As you move further away from that photo, whenever you're struggling for motivation, that photo will most likely give you the kick up the arse you need!

9. **Do your leftovers first:** And what I mean by that is, don't wait to eat then see what's leftover, serve up your meal and pack away the excess immediately. First up it makes sure you control your portion size when serving up, but also by packing them away, you're less likely to go back for more.

10. **Move the snacks out of your eye line:** There was a study on secretaries where they put snacks out on their desks. For one group they put them in plain view, and the other they put them behind something. They were around the same distance away, but the ones who couldn't see the snacks ate less of them.

11. **Get better sleep:** It's not all about how much you move to lose weight, sleeping is when your body repairs itself and makes changes. Poor sleep can not only increase your risk of cardiovascular because by 48%, but it can up your risk of obesity by 55%! So maybe turn out that light a little bit earlier from now on!

12. **Put your cutlery down:** Studies have shown that eating slower makes you feel full more quickly. It takes time for your brain's hunger signals to catch up with the food hitting your stomach, so eating fast doesn't give you a chance to do that. Try putting your knife and fork down in between mouthfuls.

13. **Go red:** If you're making a salad, add in some red cabbage. Red cabbage specifically has been shown to not only increase the production of your body's fat burners, but also it suppresses your appetite. Wesley Snipes was wrong, always bet on red!

14. **Spice up your life:** One of those unlikely fat burners hiding in your kitchen cupboards is cinnamon. Just half a teaspoon of cinnamon each day has been shown to potentially help you burn an extra 2 pounds per month! I'd probably sprinkle it on something rather than eat it from the spoon though...

15. **Check your friends:** We know that we're influenced by the people around us, but studies have shown that if we hang out with people who are obese, we're more than 60% more likely to be obese ourselves. Why is that? Because the food and lIfestyle choices they make skew what we perceive as normal. On the flipside, hanging out with people who lead a healthy lifestyle can also help you do the same. So have a look around you. Who's supportive of you and who's dragging you down? Might be time for an audit!

16. **Buddy up:** If you workout with a buddy, you'll perform better. In one study those paired with a buddy lasted 1.8 times as long. However, those who were paired with someone slightly better than them lasted over twice as long! So it pays not to work out alone.

17. **Switch out the mayo:** Mayo seems to be in everything, but 100g has nearly 700 calories! Every tablespoon adds 100 calories to your meal. Greek yoghurt on the other hand has less than 60 per 100g – and only 12 calories per tablespoon and gives a very similar effect in your sandwich.

18. **Cut back your TV:** Studies show that people who watch a lot of TV tend to be overweight. As well as sitting still for long periods, the bright colours and loud noises encourage snacking.

19. **Turn down the volume:** Speaking of which, did you know your stereo could be fattening? Loud noises produce stress chemicals in our brain that may make people overeat.

20. **Avoid loud colours at the dinner table:** Ever wonder why most restaurants have brightly coloured paintings and tablecloths? Studies have shown it's because bright colours make food look more appealing and stimulate the appetite. Stick to neutral and pastel colours at your own dinner table to avoid the excess chow.

21. **Sit straight and stand tall:** Proper posture not only makes you look immediately slimmer, taller, and more confident, it burns more calories too. When you're doing it all day long, those extra calories can add up!

22. **Drink water while working out**: Dehydrating a muscle by just 3% has been shown to decrease strength by 10%. Doesn't take much!

23. **Drink your coffee:** Drinking caffeine before exercise can increase your performance by up to 60%!

24. **Eat off blue plates:** Research has shown that eating off of plates that are the same colour as the food on them (e.g. white plates and pasta) tends to make us eat more. Blue on the other hand doesn't really match any food so can suppress our appetite.

25. **Go Greek:** Snacking on Greek yoghurt in the afternoon has been shown to reduce hunger and lower the amount you eat come dinner time. Smashing your plate is optional.

26. **Pick a meal pattern and stick to it:** Your body thrives on predictability. If it knows what's coming and better yet when, you won't trigger any fat storage survival mechanisms.

27. **Eat more fibre:** One study showed those who added extra fibre into their diet without changing anything else lost the same amount of weight as those following the Heart-Healthy eating plan. Fibre helps us feel full and adds satiety to our diets.

28. **Don't eat at your desk:** Research studying people's lunch habits showed that those who ate lunch away from their desk ate 250 fewer calories.

29. **Eat red peppers:** They contain capsaicin, the chemical that gives them their distinctive taste and which can boost your resting metabolic rate by 25%.

30. **Have a laugh:** A good strong laugh for 10-15 minutes a day increases weekly energy consumption by up to 280 calories.

Inspiration

Gail Waller

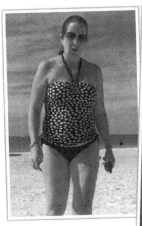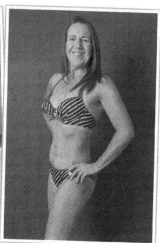

In my 20s, I was a skinny thing who could eat whatever I wanted, spend entire weekends lounging around and not put on a single pound of weight. I had no idea how lucky I was! Fast forward to my early 40s and it was an entirely different story.

I had two young boys, was working full time in a fairly demanding job and studying to become a solicitor. Although my husband and parents were all really supportive, I found that there were never enough hours in the day. I was constantly thinking about all the tasks I had to do – sorting out a costume for World Book Day, sewing on Cub badges, writing college assignments, preparing for business meetings, laundry... the list went on and on. Finding time to exercise or eat properly seemed impossible.

I realised that all my clothes were getting tighter; I didn't feel comfortable in anything. Pencil skirts for the office would cut into my stomach so I started wearing loose fitting trousers and shapeless tops. A night out with girlfriends would involve me wrestling my body into a pair of Spanx in the hope of disguising the bumps and bulges.

I told myself that there was nothing I could do. I was a busy working mum and, although I wanted to be healthy, I simply didn't have the time to prepare nutritious meals. By the time I got home from work each day, I was so shattered I just chucked a pizza in the oven or ordered a takeaway.

At a family christening, I bumped into my uncle, a former personal trainer who commented on the change in me since he'd last seen me. "Well I'm very busy, you know. I don't have time to work out!" I blurted defensively. "But you still find time to eat, don't you?" he replied and walked away. I was devastated.

In an attempt to shift the weight, I joined a local gym. I would go along on a Sunday morning and spend 10 minutes on the cross-trainer but, as soon as I got out of breath or broke a sweat, I would stop and head for the jacuzzi. None of the staff at the gym seemed bothered about how often or how long I worked out and, after a couple of months, I stopped going altogether. The gym membership would still leave my account every month and I would tell myself that I needed membership because I intended to go back. But I never did.

One day, I saw that a former colleague was checking in on Facebook to Anthony's transformation studio. She was doing it A LOT and at "silly o'clock" in the morning before I'd even rubbed the sleep from my eyes! Upon further investigation, I found that many friends and acquaintances were or had been members and all wrote really positive reviews. I noticed there was a challenge – *Drop a Dress Size in 21 Days* – and decided I'd give it a go. So I got in touch with Anthony and went in for a chat about what I wanted to achieve and how he could help me.

At first, I struggled with some of the exercises but Anthony explained that there were variations depending on ability and I could take it down a level if needed. In the first week, I got lots of emails from Anthony explaining how to cope with sore muscles and encouraging me to keep going.

Using Anthony's online meal plans and recipes, and sharing ideas with the team, I started planning and preparing meals in advance so my family was eating healthier.

At the end of the 21 day challenge, I was amazed to find that I had lost 6lb of fat and gained 2lb of muscle. My clothes were looser, and I felt much better in myself.

A few months later and I've lost over 20lbs but, to be honest, I've stopped worrying about the scales. It's about what I see in the mirror. My arms are looking toned, my legs and bum aren't wobbly anymore and I have abs! Turning up at 06.30 three times a week and spending 30 minutes doing pushups, planks, squats, lunges and crunches has paid off.

More importantly, I feel so much more energised and I can cope with the challenges of being a busy working mum. That 06.30 workout sets me up for the whole day, no matter what life throws at me.

I cannot recommend Anthony and his team of knowledgeable, friendly personal trainers highly enough. If you're looking for a fun and welcoming fitness class, at times which suit your busy lifestyle, come along and give it a try. You won't look back!

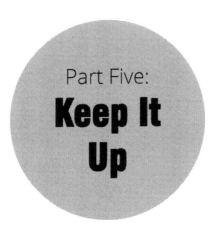

Part Five:
Keep It Up

Chapter 18

All of the Hotness,
All of the Time

*"If you're persistent, you will get it. If you're consistent, you
will keep it."*

– Jeromy Shingongo

So you've been diligently slogging away. The blood, sweat, and tears have
all been worth it, and you're happy in your own skin.

When you go shopping, you can get into pretty much whatever you fancy
without looking for things to hide those lumps and bumps you don't like.
You've thrown out the Spanx, and retired that one outfit you'd worn to
the last eleventy-million events because it was the only one you felt
comfortable in.

How do you avoid bouncing back to where you started?

Honestly, getting to this point was the hardest bit! Maintaining, or even
improving from here is pretty simple, and it's simple because you laid the
foundations getting to this point.

You didn't starve yourself, or rely on replacing meals with shakes. You didn't survive on cabbage soup, or cut entire food groups from your diet.

You ate a healthy, balanced, portion controlled diet.

You didn't sweat it out running to the moon and back every week on a treadmill. You didn't sacrifice your social life to shoehorn every class at the gym into your schedule just to burn as many calories as possible.

You threw out the notion that you need to burn as many calories as you can in the gym, and created a workout schedule that worked around your daily life, no matter how hectic it got.

So what you did was form new habits. You created a new lifestyle that runs on autopilot.

Yeah, some days it can still be difficult to drag yourself out of bed because the neighbour's dog kept you up all night. Or you might not feel like meal prepping because you got stuck in traffic on the way home and all you can think about is the butt-muppet that cut you up at the roundabout. Life's not perfect, and these things happen.

But most of the time you're all over it like hair on a Yeti because you've taken the time to become unconsciously competent.

So if you don't need to lose any more weight, maintaining your new shape is actually — you've guessed it — super simple!

Step One - Workouts

Working out to stay in shape can be approached in a couple of ways. You can keep doing exactly what you're doing, or you can step back off the throttle a little bit.

As we've discussed, your workouts aren't the big lever in your weight loss, your nutrition is. Your workouts sculpt and shape your body, but your nutrition will ultimately determine if your weight goes up or down.

So if you're happy with your workout schedule, no matter how rigid or flexible you've made it, then fill your boots! It don't need fixing, because it clearly ain't broke.

If you want to bring it down a notch, that's fine too. As long as you're getting in 2-4 workouts per week, then you'll keep a good stronghold on what you've achieved, no problem.

The other thing you can do is a combination of the too. Back off the throttle for a few weeks, then ramp it up for a few weeks. Lather, rinse, repeat. That ramp-up period could also be used to focus on a specific body part you want to nail.

Don't overthink it. As long as you're regularly getting in your MRT workouts, how and when you approach your workouts can be more flexible than a Russian gymnast.

Step Two - Nutrition

To lose weight, you'll probably be eating around 300-500 fewer calories than you need to maintain it. So to maintain your weight, guess what?

You get to eat more!

Happy days.

Again, simplicity is your friend. Add in 2-4 extra servings of protein or carbohydrates over the course of the day.

That's it!

If you find the fat is creeping on like a flabby ninja, cut back a little bit. If you find you're still losing weight, add a little bit in. As another fit-pro I know always says, "It ain't rocket surgery".

Inspiration

Val Gayes

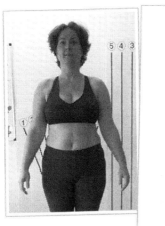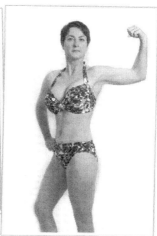

I am French born and bred, so needless to say I am naturally blessed with a healthy obsession with good food and wine. I've never been particularly overweight, never been skinny either, and never completely happy with my weight.

Since getting married, I had gradually adapted what I eat to accommodate my rather fussy eater of a husband, just to save me from cooking separate meals. Over time, this has led to compromise and laziness, and my waistline had suffered as a result. Admittedly I wasn't living on crisps and chocolate, but I was eating too much, and not enough of the good stuff.

I had tried losing weight before, mostly through starving myself (though that could never last longer than a day or two, life is just too short!), or meal replacement shakes that would never re-educate my brain and stomach about what constitutes a healthy eating lifestyle (and often contained as much sugars as a chocolate bar!) I had had some success a couple of years ago when enrolling on a personal training programme that addressed nutrition and exercise, but somehow, that didn't make a lasting change on my habits.

I had come across Anthony a few years back when he gave a talk at an event I attended, and he seemed to know his stuff about food and exercise. When I saw an advert for his personal training programme, I emailed a few questions and quickly signed up in cold blood. My mind was set, I was ready to do something about "it".

My battle was fought mostly in the kitchen. I started by weighing every meal ingredient, which was a real eye opener. For the first week, I kept wondering where was the second half of my meals... I'd pretty much been eating for two. My brain would try to convince me I needed more so I started to drink more water and green tea. Coconut oil and snacks of biltong became my new friends.

I printed off every single download I could find on Anthony's website – All the meal plans, the nutrition manual, the recipes – and I put everything in a big folder that I studied like a geek and took action. To start with, I struggled with guilt for letting my husband sort his dinners out but concluded I was doing what was right for me.

I don't have a natural love of exercise, so the workouts were not particularly enjoyable to start with, but my mind was made that I was just going to turn up, do as I was told and go home. I would not let my mind talk me out of it, and soon, two training sessions a week became the norm. I threw in a yoga class too for good measure.

I was setting up good habits and the weight was falling off. Not super fast, but I was after a life change, not a quick fix. I'd already tried the quick fixes, it was time to do it right!

I dropped 44 lbs over about 9 months, that's around 1.5 lbs a week, I'm happy with that. I've gone from a near UK size 16 to a nearly size 10, and had to punch an extra 11 holes in my belt. I've dropped all my "Excess" body fat, going from just over 30% body fat to just under 17%.

And it hasn't been as hard as I thought it might be. The most important factor in my success was deciding from the start that I wanted to do this.

My attitude to food has changed too. It's no longer used as a source of comfort, but as a source of nourishment for my body. I eat well and exercise because I want to look after the body I have now, not necessarily because I am aiming for the perfect body (whatever that is?!) And if I go away for the weekend, or have the odd meal out, I don't agonise over what to eat, I just enjoy it!

I'm thankful for all the help, encouragement and knowledge I have been given by Anthony and his team. There's a real community and family feel, and we all seem to be rooting for each other. I definitely found myself in good company!

About the Author

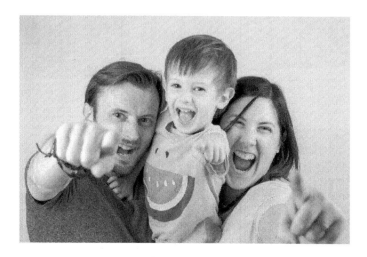

Hi, I'm Anthony...

Family man. Father. Tea addict. Pun lover. David Tennant lookalike. But not professionally...

I was going to give you the standard clinical, "I'm a fitness Trainer, and I'm certified with several different governing bodies, have over 20 years' experience whipping people into shape, and have had training programmes used by magazines such as Men's Health, blah, blah, blah..." on this page.

However, while that is true – I do have over 20 years' experience, hold more fitness qualifications than I care to count, and so on – to be honest, that doesn't really tell you anything about me.

See, a lot of trainers fall into their vocation because they're naturally fit. As a result, they only need stick on a vest and some shorts and you'll immediately believe anything they say. Unfortunately, despite qualifications, they tend to think that what works for them (which is most things) will work for everyone else!

That's not me though. Quite the opposite, in fact.

As a teenager, I weighed 7 stone. Problem was, as we moved further into our teenage years, everyone around me seemed to be getting bigger, stronger, more athletic... and I didn't! The muscle building, fat burning effects of puberty seemed to completely pass me by.

I quickly decided I didn't want to be at the back of the pack, and started learning about working out. Unfortunately, I did it the wrong way by picking up fitness mags and following what the models and trainers in those told me to do.

What I didn't realise was that the people in those mags were naturally in that shape. They gained easy, and 95% of their shape came from what their parents gave them. People like you and me need to put in months of effort just to look like their "before" photo!

Years later and into my 20s, I'd managed to build myself up to a whopping 8 and a half stone. Great! (I say that sarcastically, but as someone who used to weigh just 7 stone, it actually was for me!)

When I finally ditched the fitness mags and hit the real books, I became incredibly intimate with the inner workings of the human body.

I learned, picked up several qualifications along the way, and as I did, it was only then I started seeing real results. Had I not spent countless hours studying, practicing, and just getting myself out there in the trenches, I would never have reached a point where I'm happy to wear clothes that fit when it's hot, and not sweat it out in something long and baggy to hide my embarrassment!

I then went on to create transformation programmes for average Joes and Janes, just like me, and the results I was getting started to get noticed.

I was head-hunted by national magazines.

I was asked to put readers through my programmes. To write new, unique programmes to get people the kind of results you normally only see if you're a movie star. But somewhere along the way, disaster jumped up and kicked me in the man-berries. Or the lower back to be more precise.

I never had a coach. I learned exercise form from books with no-one to keep an eye on me and make sure I'm not going to hurt myself... But I did!

One day in the gym, while squatting with way too much weight on my shoulders and, shall we say, questionable form, something 'went' in my lower back. For years I was plagued with chronic pain whenever I tried to do any kind of exercise. I took a few steps forward then a few back, and eventually after years on the NHS hamster wheel, I gave in and paid to get proper physio.

This worked great, finally allowing me to train properly, and let me make real progress.

Up until I became a father.

A long labour and a week sleeping in a hospital chair pushed my lower back over the edge, finally prolapsing a disc in my spine.

This left me completely twisted up, and over the next few months I piled on the fat. I was walking with a crutch and on enough pain killers and anti-inflamatories to open up a pop-up pharmacy

I ended up having to have hospital procedures, and put myself into intensive physio to get back to even walking normally again!

The silver lining to all of this is that during recovery, when I was getting back in shape I had to adapt my training, and stumbled on even faster ways to drop fat, tighten and tone, and get stronger, fitter, and healthier.

So what does that tell you about me?

I'm human. I'm vulnerable. I've failed (a lot!), and I've been broken.

I've been painfully skinny, I've been so fat I look like I've swallowed a beach-ball, and I've been everything in between.

I wasn't born in shape. I don't have the genetics to just look at a dumbbell and drop fat like a hot stone.

I understand body transformation intimately. I've lived it and do it every day.

And now I help other people get real results. In fact, at the time of writing, I've helped thousands of people slash their body fat and tone and shape their muscles through my courses, books, articles, and of course in-person training and consultations.

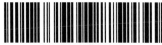

Printed in Great Britain
by Amazon